The Athlete's Elbow

Guest Editor

MARC R. SAFRAN, MD

CLINICS IN SPORTS MEDICINE

www.sportsmed.theclinics.com

Consulting Editor
MARK D. MILLER, MD

October 2010 • Volume 29 • Number 4

SAUNDERS an imprint of ELSEVIER, Inc.

W.B. SAUNDERS COMPANY

A Division of Elsevier Inc.

1600 John F. Kennedy Blvd. • Suite 1800 • Philadelphia, Pennsylvania 19103

http://www.theclinics.com

CLINICS IN SPORTS MEDICINE Volume 29, Number 4
October 2010 ISSN 0278-5919, ISBN-13: 978-1-4377-2498-1

Editor: Ruth Malwitz
Developmental Editor: Jessica Demetriou

Clinics in Sports Medicine (ISSN 0278-5919) is published quarterly by Elsevier Inc., 360 Park Avenue South, New York, NY 10010-1710. Months of issue are January, April, July, and October. Business and Editorial Offices: 1600 John F. Kennedy Blvd., Ste. 1800, Philadelphia, PA 19103-2899. Customer Service Office: 3251 Riverport Lane, Maryland Heights, MO 63043. Periodicals postage paid at New York, NY and additional mailing offices. Subscription prices are $297.00 per year (US individuals), $466.00 per year (US institutions), $147.00 per year (US students), $337.00 per year (Canadian individuals), $563.00 per year (Canadian institutions), $205.00 (Canadian students), $409.00 per year (foreign individuals), $563.00 per year (foreign institutions), and $205.00 per year (foreign students). Foreign air speed delivery is included in all *Clinics* subscription prices. All prices are subject to change without notice. **POSTMASTER:** Send address changes to *Clinics in Sports Medicine*, Elsevier Health Sciences Division, Subscription Customer Service, 3251 Riverport Lane, Maryland Heights, MO 63043. Customer Service (orders, claims, online, change of address): Elsevier Health Sciences Division, Subscription Customer Service, 3251 Riverport Lane, Maryland Heights, MO 63043. Tel: 1-800-654-2452 (U.S. and Canada); 314-447-8871 (outside U.S. and Canada). Fax: 314-447-8029. E-mail: journalscustomerservice-usa@elsevier.com (for print support); journalsonlinesupport-usa@elsevier.com (for online support).

Reprints. For copies of 100 or more of articles in this publication, please contact the Commercial Reprints Department, Elsevier Inc., 360 Park Avenue South, New York, NY 10010-1710. Tel.: 212-633-3812; Fax: 212-462-1935; E-mail: reprints@elsevier.com.

Clinics in Sports Medicine is covered in *MEDLINE/PubMed (Index Medicus) Current Contents/Clinical Medicine, Excerpta Medica,* and *ISI/Biomed.*

Printed and bound in the United Kingdom
Transferred to Digital Print 2011

Contributors

CONSULTING EDITOR

MARK D. MILLER, MD
S. Ward Casscells Professor of Orthopaedic Surgery, University of Virginia, Charlottesville, Virginia; Team Physician, James Madison University, Harrisonburg, Virginia

GUEST EDITOR

MARC R. SAFRAN, MD
Professor, Department of Orthopaedic Surgery; Associate Director, Sports Medicine, Stanford University, California

AUTHORS

CHRISTOPHER S. AHMAD, MD
Associate Professor, Department of Orthopaedic Surgery, Columbia University Medical center, New York, New York

GREGORY I. BAIN, MBBS, FRACS, PhD
Senior Visiting Orthopaedic Surgeon, Orthopaedic Department, Modbury Hospital, Modbury; Department of Orthopaedic Surgery, University of Adelaide, Royal Adelaide Hospital, South Australia, Australia

CHAMP L. BAKER Jr, MD, FACS
Staff Physician, The Hughston Foundation; The Hughston Clinic, Columbus; Department of Orthopaedic Surgery, Medical College of Georgia, Augusta, Georgia

CHAMP L. BAKER III, MD
Staff Physician, The Hughston Foundation; The Hughston Clinic, Columbus, Georgia

JEFFREY R. DUGAS, MD
American Sports Medicine Institute, Birmingham, Alabama

ADAM W. DURRANT, MB, ChB, FRACS
Senior Visiting Orthopaedic Surgeon, Orthopaedic Department, Modbury Hospital, Modbury; Department of Orthopaedic Surgery, University of Adelaide, Royal Adelaide Hospital, South Australia, Australia

TODD S. ELLENBECKER, DPT, MS, SCS, OCS, CSCS
Clinic Director, Physiotherapy Associates, Scottsdale Sports Clinic, Scottsdale, Arizona; National Director Of Clinical Research, Physiotherapy Associates, Exton, Pennsylvania; Director of Sports Medicine, ATP World Tour, Florida

LARRY D. FIELD, MD
Director, Upper Extremity Service, Mississippi Sports Medicine and Orthopaedic Center; Clinical Associate Professor, Department of Orthopaedic Surgery, University of Mississippi Medical School, Jackson, Mississippi

R. MICHAEL GREIWE, MD
Fellow, Shoulder, Elbow, and Sports Medicine, Department of Orthopaedic Surgery, Columbia University Medical Center, New York, New York

DANIEL J. GURLEY, MD
College Park Family Care Center, Kansas City, Kansas

SANAZ HARIRI, MD
Fellow, Sports Medicine, Department of Orthopaedic Surgery, Stanford University, Menlo Park, California

TIMOTHY R. MCADAMS, MD
Associate Professor, Orthopaedic Surgery, Stanford University, Redwood City, California

EUGENE G. MCNALLY, MD, FRCR
Consultant Musculoskeletal Radiologist, Nuffield Orthopaedic Centre, Oxford, United Kingdom

CORY O. NELSON, MD
Sports Medicine and Arthroscopic Surgery, Spine & Orthopedic Specialists, Scottsdale, Arizona

MICHAEL J. O'BRIEN, MD
Assistant Professor, Department of Orthopaedic Surgery, Tulane University, New Orleans, Louisiana

BRADFORD O. PARSONS, MD
Assistant Professor, Department of Orthopaedic Surgery, Mount Sinai School of Medicine, New York, New York

MATTHEW L. RAMSEY, MD
Shoulder and Elbow Service, Rothman Institute; Associate Professor of Orthopaedic Surgery, Thomas Jefferson University, Philadelphia, Pennsylvania

MICHAEL REINOLD, DPT, SCS, ATC, CSCS
Boston Red Sox Baseball Club, Division of Sports Medicine, Department of Orthopaedic Surgery, Massachusetts General Hospital, Boston, Massachusetts

MARC R. SAFRAN, MD
Professor, Department of Orthopaedic Surgery; Associate Director, Sports Medicine, Stanford University, California

COMRON SAIFI, MS
Research Assistant, Department of Orthopaedic Surgery, Columbia University Medical Center, New York, New York

FELIX H. SAVOIE III, MD
Lee C. Schlesinger Professor, Department of Orthopaedic Surgery; Director, Tulane Institute of Sports Medicine, Tulane University, New Orleans, Louisiana

KATHRYN J. STEVENS, MD, FRCR
Associate Professor of Radiology, Department of Radiology, Stanford University Medical Center, Stanford University School of Medicine, Stanford, California

CHRISTOPHER VAN HOFWEGEN, MD
Fellow in Sports Medicine, The Hughston Foundation, Columbus, Georgia; Bellingham, Washington

Contents

Acute and chronic elbow pain is common, particularly in athletes. Although plain radiographs, ultrasound, and computed tomography all have a role to play in the investigation of elbow pain, magnetic resonance imaging (MRI) has emerged as the imaging modality of choice for diagnosis of soft tissue disease and osteochondral injury around the elbow. The high spatial resolution, excellent soft-tissue contrast, and multiplanar imaging capabilities of MRI make it ideal for evaluating the complex joint anatomy of the elbow. This article reviews imaging of common disease conditions occurring around the elbow in athletes, with an emphasis on MRI.

Biceps or triceps ruptures are rare but can cause a significant disability. Surgical repair has become the preferred method of treatment for the complete rupture, but the decision when to treat partial tears is less clear. Reconstruction of the tendon is the preferred method when patients have a delayed presentation.

Epicondylitis is a diagnostic term that describes a pattern of pain and tenderness localized to the medial or lateral epicondyles of the distal humerus. The pathoanatomy, clinical presentation, and treatment of these disorders is described. Nonoperative treatment, operative techniques, postoperative care, and the results of treatment are discussed.

Elbow dislocation in the athletic population is not an uncommon injury. The literature does not clearly establish treatment guidelines, with treatment being extrapolated from the experience in the general population. A short period of immobilization with early range of motion exercises limits disability and allows return to sports participation within 6 weeks.

pain and dysfunction. Both of these conditions are treated initially with rest from throwing, followed by gradual return to throwing through an interval throwing program. When conservative measures fail, minimally invasive or arthroscopic surgical procedures can be used to address the problem. Successful return to competitive overhead sports is expected at all levels of competition with these conditions.

Nerve Injuries About the Elbow

Sanaz Hariri and Timothy R. McAdams

The ulnar, radial, median, medial antebrachial cutaneous, and lateral ante-brachial cutaneous nerves are subject to traction and compression in athletes who place forceful, repetitive stresses across their elbow joint. Throwing athletes are at greatest risk, and cubital tunnel syndrome (involving the ulnar nerve) is clearly the most common neuropathy about the elbow. The anatomy and innervation pattern of the nerve involved determines the characteristic of the neuropathy syndrome. The most important parts of the work-up are the history and physical examination as electro-diagnostic testing and imaging are often not reliable. In general, active rest is the first line of treatment. Tailoring the surgery and rehabilitation protocol according to the functional requirements of that athlete's sport(s) can help optimize the operative outcomes for recalcitrant cases.

Pediatric Sports Elbow Injuries

R. Michael Greiwe, Comron Saifi, and Christopher S. Ahmad

Elbow injuries in the pediatric and adolescent population represent a spectrum of pathology that can be categorized as medial tension injuries, lateral compression injuries, and posterior shear injuries. Early and accurate diagnosis can improve outcomes for both nonoperative and operative treatments. Prevention strategies are important to help reduce the increasing incidence of elbow injuries in youth athletes.

Clinical Concepts for Treatment of the Elbow in the Adolescent Overhead Athlete

Todd S. Ellenbecker, Michael Reinold, and Cory O. Nelson

Injuries to the adolescent elbow are common because of the repetitive overuse inherent in many overhead sport activities. The management of these patients is greatly facilitated through a greater understanding of the demands placed on the upper extremity kinetic chain during these overhead activities as well as a detailed examination and rehabilitation for the entire upper extremity kinetic chain. Particular emphasis on improving rotator cuff strength and muscular endurance, along with scapular stabilization, is a critical part of elbow rehabilitation in these patients. In addition, the use of a strategic and progressive interval sport return program is necessary to minimize reinjury and return the adolescent overhead athlete to full function.

THE CLINICS ARE NOW AVAILABLE ONLINE!

Access your subscription at:
www.theclinics.com

Foreword

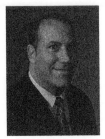

Mark D. Miller, MD
Consulting Editor

It is hard to believe that it has been 7 to 8 years since I first asked my friend and colleague, Dr Marc Safran, to guest edit an edition of *Clinics in Sports Medicine* dedicated to the athlete's elbow. Although we both completed the same fellowship, my interest in elbow surgery waned, and his interest blossomed. I suspect that a lot of that is because we have very talented elbow surgeons at my University, and much of that fell to Dr Safran at his institution.

It is equally hard to believe how much elbow surgery has advanced in those same 7 to 8 years. In fact, I did not even know what "VEOS" (Dugas article) even was (valgus extension overload syndrome) until I consulted with our elbow surgeons and read Dr Safran's Preface.

I have asked Dr Safran to participate in a number of projects in recent years, and I doubt that he will agree to do a third update in 7 to 8 more years because he will still be working on our current mutual projects! Nevertheless, I am very pleased that this issue turned out so well and am honored to expose you, the reader, to his talents!

This is a thorough treatise on elbow injuries in the athlete. It is well organized, beginning with imaging and ending with rehabilitation, and includes a complete discussion of key sports-related elbow conditions in between. There is a veritable Who's Who list of contributors, and we should all be grateful for that. This is truly an outstanding edition. Enjoy!

Mark D. Miller, MD
Department of Orthopaedic Surgery
University of Virginia
400 Ray C. Hunt Drive, Suite 330
Charlottesville, VA 22908-0159, USA

E-mail address:
mdm3p@virginia.edu

Clin Sports Med 29 (2010) xi
doi:10.1016/j.csm.2010.06.003
0278-5919/10/$ – see front matter © 2010 Elsevier Inc. All rights reserved.

Preface

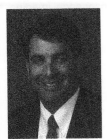

Marc R. Safran, MD
Guest Editor

There continues to be increasing interest focused on the athletic elbow. Since my last issue for *Clinics in Sports Medicine* on elbow injuries in athletes in 2004, there continues to be a growing interest in the evaluation and management of elbow injuries in the active population. This interest is being accompanied by increasing research of elbow function, mechanics, and pathomechanics, as is reflected by the expanding body of literature about elbow injuries. As we move forward, there are more new diagnostic tools and greater awareness of these injuries, which is fueling the interest by identifying a significant and increasing incidence of athletic elbow injuries, which may be affected by intrinsic as well as extrinsic factors. Outcomes studies are helping define optimal treatment techniques for elbow maladies, which, in conjunction with better and reproducible surgical results, are stimulating clinician interest in identifying these problems. Elbow injuries in athletes are certainly performance as well as potentially career issues. As such, proper identification and management of these problems are of paramount importance. With the recent advances in clinical outcomes, it is timely to publish this issue of *Clinics in Sports Medicine* as an update to the previous issue. The goal was to compile and summarize the most current knowledge and state-of-the-art information by many of the world's experts about elbow injuries in athletes to update the sports medicine physician, including hot topics like platelet rich plasma.

This issue of *Clinics in Sports Medicine* is written and compiled with the sports physician in mind. It is written about elbow injuries in the high level competitive athlete as well as the recreational athlete. Some injuries, such as injury to the ulnar collateral ligament, occur much more frequently in the athlete; however, many of these problems, such as lateral epicondylitis and biceps tendon ruptures, occur more frequently in those not participating in high school, collegiate, or professional sports. No matter whether these injuries occur in the computer jockey, motocross rider, golfer, or baseball pitcher, it is the sports medicine physician that is usually called on to manage these elbow injuries. It was with this thought in mind that this issue of *Clinics* was compiled.

Clin Sports Med 29 (2010) xiii–xv
doi:10.1016/j.csm.2010.06.002   **sportsmed.theclinics.com**
0278-5919/10/$ – see front matter © 2010 Elsevier Inc. All rights reserved.

In the first article, a collaborative effort by Dr Stevens, my radiology partner at Stanford, and Dr McNally from Oxford, England, a comprehensive review of the imaging of the elbow is presented. While concentrating on magnetic resonance imaging, they also discuss plain radiographs and the role of ultrasonography of the elbow with excellent case examples.

Clinically, starting with musculotendinous problems about the elbow, two excellent articles are provided. First, Drs Bain and Durrant from Australia review distal biceps' and triceps anatomy and injury, as well as treatment. Dr Bain has contributed extensively to the literature with his original work about the anatomy of the distal biceps, as well as tenoscopy and endobutton repair of the distal biceps, making this an appropriate topic for him to review. Next, Dr Champ Baker Jr with Drs Van Hofwegen and Champ Baker III, from the Hughston Clinic, review the etiology, evaluation, and management medial and lateral epicondylitis of the elbow. This article includes the long term perspective of Dr Baker's innovation of arthroscopic management tennis elbow as well as the management of medial epicondylitis. This article also reviews some of the current hot topics in sports medicine, such as PRP.

Next are a series of articles on elbow ligamentous injuries. Drs Matthew Ramsey of the Rothman Institute in Philadelphia and Dr Bradford Parsons of Mt Sinai School of Medicine in New York review the current management of acute elbow dislocations. This is an up-to-date review of this common elbow malady that has recent changes in thought about management. Following this is an interesting article with new and original thoughts about the management of posterolateral rotatory instability, usually a consequence of elbow dislocation. Drs Savoie, O'Brien, Field, and Gurley review the arthroscopic and open management of radio-ulnohumeral ligament reconstruction for posterolateral rotatory instability, discussing new open techniques to better reconstruct the true pathology, as well as the indications, technique, and results of arthroscopic lateral ligament plication. The last article in this section is a review of ulnar collateral ligament injury in the overhead athlete, including a discussion of the secondary changes that occur from repeated valgus stress to the elbow by Dr Hariri and me. The biomechanics, history, physical examination, and ancillary tests are discussed, in addition to the treatment of ulnar collateral ligament injury in the thrower's elbow.

Dr Dugas from the American Sports Medicine Institute in Birmingham, Alabama, a sports medicine center that treats many overhead athletes, particularly baseball players, reviews the diagnosis and treatment of posterior compartment elbow injuries. In addition to valgus extension overload, this article includes their thoughts on stress fractures of the olecranon, and arthroscopy of the posterior compartment of the elbow. Drs Hariri and McAdams, my partner at Stanford, a Team Physician for the San Francisco 49ers and fellowship-trained hand surgeon, extensively review the etiology, presentation, evaluation, and management of common nerve lesions about the elbow in athletes. They provide many useful tables and figures to simplify this complex topic.

In the next article, Dr Ahmad leads an authorship team of Drs Greiwe and Saifi from Columbia University in New York reviewing various common pediatric athletic elbow injuries. Dr Ahmad, team physician for the New York Yankees, has a special interest in pediatric sports medicine, giving him a unique perspective on pediatric sports elbow injuries. This article begins with the latest information on the understanding of the throwing mechanics in children as compared with adults. They review medial-sided injuries, such as apophysitis, medial epicondyle avulsion injuries, and ulnar collateral ligament injuries, in youth. Laterally, they review Panner's disease; also, an excellent comprehensive review of osteochondritis dissecans and the newest thoughts on its management, in addition to tennis elbow and radiocapitellar plica, are presented.

Finally, they review posterior compartment injuries, such as olecranon apophyseal injuries and stress fractures, and discuss elbow injury prevention.

The last article was written by a trio of experts in elbow rehabilitation: Todd Ellenbecker, a physical therapist who is the Director of Sports Medicine for the ATP (Association of Tennis Professionals—the men's professional tennis tour) as well as the Head of the Sports Science Committee for the USTA (United States Tennis Association), the National Director of Clinical Research for Physiotherapy Associates, and Clinic Director of the Physiotherapy Associates Scottsdale, Arizona clinic; Michael Reinold, a physical therapist and head athletic trainer for the Boston Red Sox Baseball club; and Dr Corey Nelson, a sports medicine orthopedic surgeon in Scottsdale, Arizona. This article provides some interesting cutting edge thoughts about clinical concepts in the treatment of the elbow in the adolescent overhead athlete, focusing on baseball and tennis.

Great care and effort has been put forth by the authors in compiling this edition of *Clinics in Sports Medicine.* As increasing attention is being paid to the elbow in athletes, this edition of *Clinics in Sports Medicine* provides the most current, state-of-the-art information to the clinician, written by many leaders in this field. The end result is what I and the contributing authors would hope to be a useful, comprehensive, and up-to-date review of elbow injuries in athletes.

Marc R. Safran, MD
Sports Medicine, Department of Orthopaedic Surgery
Stanford University
450 Broadway Street, M/C 6342
Redwood City, CA 94063, USA

E-mail address:
msafran@stanford.edu

Magnetic Resonance Imaging of the Elbow in Athletes

Kathryn J. Stevens, MD, FRCR[a],*, Eugene G. McNally, MD, FRCR[b]

KEYWORDS

- Elbow • MRI • Ligaments • Tendons • Nerve
- Bursitis • Osteochondral

Elbow pain is a commonly presenting symptom in athletes, particularly those involved in overhead throwing sports such as tennis, cricket, baseball, and javelin, and in golf. The elbow can be injured acutely by either direct trauma or as a result of forces transmitted to the elbow by a fall on an outstretched hand. Chronic repetitive stress can also affect structures around the elbow, producing symptoms that may be extremely debilitating and disruptive for high-level athletes.

IMAGING MODALITIES
Radiography

Plain radiographs are recommended as the investigation of choice after an acute injury to the elbow to determine if there is soft tissue swelling, a joint effusion, or visible bony injury. In a more chronic setting, radiographs may also detect soft tissue calcification, enthesopathic change, bone spurs, or advanced osteochondral disease. A standard trauma series consists of anteroposterior (AP) and lateral radiographs of the elbow, with the addition of 2 oblique views in internal and external rotation as clinically indicated. A joint effusion can be detected radiographically by the displacement of lucent fat pads from the coronoid and olecranon fossae. The anterior fat pad is normally visible on a lateral radiograph (**Fig. 1**), but becomes triangular or sail-shaped in the presence of a joint effusion, producing the anterior fat pad sign (**Fig. 2**). The posterior fat pad is seen only if a joint effusion is present (see **Fig. 2**), so therefore its detection is a more reliable assessment of acute effusion. With chronic effusion and, in particular more long-standing synovial disease, the fat pad becomes infiltrated and may not be discerned from the surrounding soft tissues. If a joint effusion is apparent in an elbow following trauma but no fracture can be detected

[a] Department of Radiology, Stanford University Medical Center, Stanford University School of Medicine, Room S-062A Grant Building, 300 Pasteur Drive, Stanford, CA 94305-5105, USA
[b] Nuffield Orthopaedic Centre, Windmill Road, Headington, Oxford OX3 7LD, UK
* Corresponding author.
E-mail address: kate.stevens@stanford.edu

Clin Sports Med 29 (2010) 521–553
doi:10.1016/j.csm.2010.06.004
0278-5919/10/$ – see front matter © 2010 Elsevier Inc. All rights reserved.

sportsmed.theclinics.com

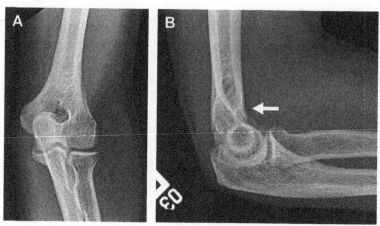

Fig. 1. (A) AP and (B) lateral radiographs of a normal elbow. A normal anterior fat pad (*arrow*) is visible on the lateral view.

radiographically, the patient is often treated as if a fracture is present, with follow-up radiographs as indicated. However, in a high-level athlete, cross-sectional imaging with computed tomography (CT) or magnetic resonance imaging (MRI) may be used to look for an occult fracture.

Stress radiographs with applied valgus or varus stress may occasionally be of help in the evaluation of ligamentous tears and joint stability, although these may be painful for the patient. For this reason stress views can also be performed in the operating room with a fluoroscopy unit once the patient is anesthetized.

Ultrasound

Ultrasound is commonly used in the evaluation of soft tissue disease around the elbow, enabling high-resolution imaging of superficial structures such as tendons, ligaments, and nerves.[1] Ultrasound is widely available, and is relatively cheap

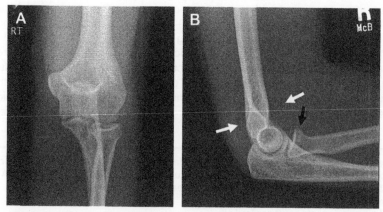

Fig. 2. (A) AP and (B) lateral radiographs of the elbow after a fall on an outstretched hand. Vague sclerosis is seen across the radial neck on the AP view. On the lateral view there is elevation of the anterior and posterior fat pads (*white arrows*), and a cortical break is seen at the radial head/neck junction (*black arrow*).

compared with CT and MRI. Many ultrasound manufacturers now make small portable machines, which gives team physicians potentially immediate access to imaging after an athlete is injured. However, such equipment rarely has the same spatial resolution and imaging quality as high-end equipment. Ultrasound can be used to detect joint effusions (**Fig. 3**), and ligamentous or tendon tears. Advantages of ultrasound include that the contralateral arm can be easily evaluated for comparison, and that the examination can be performed while moving the joint under interrogation. This method may give additional information such as the degree of tendon retraction or associated fractures, which can subsequently be used to aid surgical planning. Dynamic ultrasound can also be used to assess for pathologic conditions that may only be apparent when the limb is moved, such as ulnar nerve subluxation or muscle hernias. Ultrasound has the ability to detect subtle calcification or foreign bodies that may not be apparent on radiography (**Fig. 4**) or MRI. Ultrasound is less useful for the evaluation of deeper structures or osteochondral disease. Like MRI, musculoskeletal ultrasound also requires additional specialist training to gain maximum benefit from the technology. Furthermore, musculoskeletal ultrasound is also extremely operator dependent. Like clinical examination, it may be difficult to interpret an ultrasound examination performed by another individual, or determine whether their study is both adequate and accurate because ultrasound examinations are not always reproducible. Technological developments, including panoramic imaging, video storage, and three-dimensional (3D) probes, help to bridge the gap between stored static ultrasound and MR images.

CT

CT is widely used in the evaluation of fractures around joints to show intraarticular extension or small fracture fragments within the joint. Iodinated contrast can be given intravenously to determine whether major blood vessels adjacent to the joint are

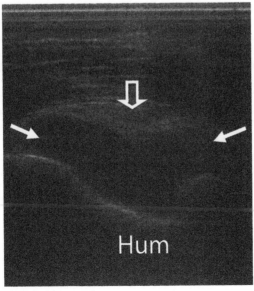

Fig. 3. Ultrasound image through the posterior elbow in the presence of a joint effusion, showing hypoechoic fluid within the olecranon fossa (*arrow*) displacing the echogenic posterior fat pad (*open arrow*).

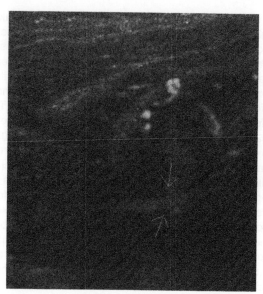

Fig. 4. Ultrasound image of the elbow in a patient with a fragment of nonradiopaque cactus thorn in the anterior joint indicated by arrows. The piece of thorn is surrounded by hypoechoic synovitis, with increased flow on color Doppler.

injured. Modern CT scanners provide excellent spatial and contrast resolution. Images are usually acquired axially, with subsequent reformation in the sagittal and coronal planes. However, images can also be reconstructed in any arbitrary oblique plane that best shows complex joint anatomy. 3D models can also be constructed from the raw data, which are helpful for surgical planning. CT is usually readily available, and close to the emergency room. Modern multislice CT scanners can perform a comprehensive examination of a joint within seconds, which minimizes motion artifact on the scan, and limits the amount of time that a sick patient has to spend in the examination room. CT may detect soft tissue calcification, myositis ossificans, and intraarticular bodies more readily than MRI. Osteoarthritis is readily apparent when the subchondral bone is involved. CT arthrography with intraarticular injection of iodinated contrast is an excellent method of detecting disease in the overlying articular cartilage, although internal structural changes are not detected if the cartilage surface is intact (**Fig. 5**). CT arthrography may be helpful if the patient has contraindications to an MRI scan, such as an intracranial aneurysm clip, pacemaker, or intraorbital metal fragments. CT arthrography has been used to evaluate the ulnar collateral ligament (UCL).[2–4] Disadvantages of CT include the resultant radiation dose, which may be a consideration if multiple examinations are necessary or if a patient is pregnant. CT also has poor soft tissue characterization, which can make detection of subtle soft tissue injuries challenging. Metallic hardware within the bones or periarticular soft tissues can cause significant beam-hardening artifact, which limits evaluation of the surrounding bone and soft tissues. Although this effect can be minimized by altering scan parameters, this can result in a larger radiation dose to the patient.

MRI

MRI, with its high spatial resolution, excellent soft tissue contrast, and multiplanar imaging capabilities, has emerged as the imaging modality of choice for the evaluation

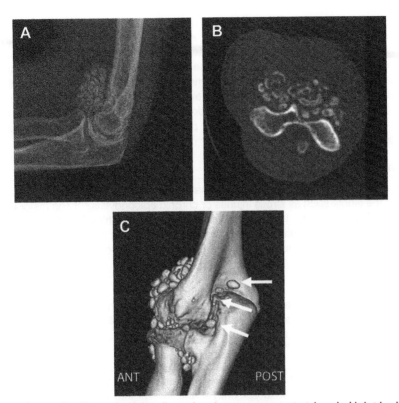

Fig. 5. (*A*) Lateral radiograph of the elbow showing numerous osteochondral joint bodies in the coronoid fossa compatible with primary synovial osteochondromatosis. (*B*) On an axial CT section, a joint body is also seen in the olecranon fossa. (*C*) A posterior oblique 3D reconstruction image shows several small joint bodies around the posterolateral elbow (*arrows*).

of elbow pain in the athlete. The patient can be scanned in either the supine or prone position, depending on the presenting symptoms, patient preference, and body habitus. It is beneficial to position a skin marker over the site of maximal symptoms, commonly consisting of a cod liver oil capsule held in place with tape. If the patient is imaged supine, the arm is positioned at their side, with a high-resolution surface coil secured in place. The supine position is the most comfortable for the patient and results in minimal motion artifact. However, the elbow is not within the isocenter of the magnet, which can result in a nonuniform magnetic field and inhomogeneous fat saturation. This position may not be possible in larger patients, and patients can be also be imaged prone with the arm extended over the head. This position places the elbow in the center of the bore, enabling uniform fat suppression. However, the prone position is uncomfortable and may be difficult to maintain for a prolonged period, making the scan susceptible to motion artifact. MRI gives excellent visualization of soft tissue and bony disease, and is able to detect subtle pathologic conditions such as bone marrow edema in an early stress injury, not apparent on radiographs or CT. MR arthrography with intraarticular injection of saline or dilute gadolinium may be helpful in patients without a joint effusion to look for subtle ligament tears, osteochondral disease, or joint bodies.[4–6] Major disadvantages of MRI include the high cost of the examination and long scan times. However, with the advent of high-field MRI scanners, scan times and image resolution have improved. MRI cannot be performed easily in patients who are claustrophobic, and oral or intravenous sedation may be necessary. Open MRI units can provide reasonable images and are certainly useful in the evaluation of bone or tendon disease. However, more subtle ligament injuries are best appreciated on higher-field systems. MRI is also contraindicated in patients who have certain implanted medical devices, such as pacemakers or nerve stimulators, or who have metal in high-risk locations such as intracranial aneurysm clips. MRI can also be challenging in obese patients, or in patients with implanted orthopedic hardware.

Radionuclide Scintigraphy

Radionuclide bone scintigraphy is occasionally used for detection of pathologic conditions of the elbow such as stress injuries or chronic epicondylitis.[7–9] The major disadvantage of a bone scan is the radiation dose incurred, which is less desirable in a younger athletic population. Bone scans are sensitive but have a poor specificity, usually necessitating further imaging if an abnormality is detected.

LIGAMENTOUS INJURIES

The ulnar and lateral collateral ligaments are the primary stabilizers of the elbow, and are commonly injured in athletes, either as a result of a single traumatic event or chronic repetitive microtrauma.

UCL

The UCL is divided into 3 bundles: anterior, posterior, and transverse. The anterior bundle arises from the medial epicondyle and inserts into the sublime tubercle of the proximal ulna, providing the principle restraint to valgus stress at the elbow. The anterior bundle itself can be further subdivided into 2 functionally separate anterior and posterior bands,[10,11] which are believed to function in a reciprocal fashion, but cannot be distinguished as 2 separate structures on imaging. The anterior bundle of the UCL is readily depicted on either MRI or ultrasound (**Fig. 6**). On MRI the proximal fibers can appear lax and slightly indistinct or splayed, and this should not be mistaken for a partial tear.[12] The ulnar attachment of the anterior bundle is usually described as inserting within 1 mm of the articular margin of the coronoid process.[13] However, a more recent article suggests that the distal insertion can be up to 3 mm distal to the sublime tubercle of the ulna.[14] This characteristic may create a small recess on MR arthrography, which can simulate a partial undersurface tear. The posterior bundle of the UCL arises from the inferior aspect of the medial epicondyle and inserts at the posteromedial margin of the trochlear notch. Although the posterior bundle can be identified on coronal images, it is best seen on axial images, in which it forms the floor of the cubital tunnel.[15] The transverse bundle bridges the ulnar insertions of the anterior and posterior bundles, is not functionally significant, and cannot be seen readily on MRI.

The anterior bundle of the UCL is amenable to ultrasound assessment. The examination is best performed with the patient seated opposite the examiner. The affected arm is placed on the examination couch and the probe is positioned over the medial aspect of the joint. The coronal plane is the best one for examining the ligament in the long axis, and 20° to 30° flexion is used to help with visualization. The normal UCL is depicted as a well-organized, predominantly reflective structure. The collagen fibers are seen as low reflective structures against a background of more reflective matrix. Complete rupture of the UCL results in disorganization of this normal structure and

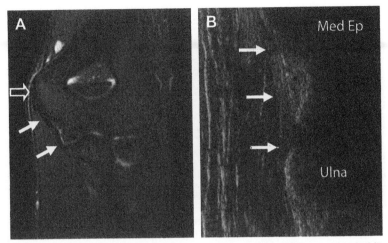

Fig. 6. Normal appearance of the MCL on MRI and ultrasound. (*A*) On a coronal oblique T2-weighted image, the anterior bundle appears as a thin band of low signal intensity extending from the medial epicondyle to the sublime tubercle, just deep to the common flexor tendon (*arrow*). (*B*) On coronal ultrasound the UCL is seen as a linear reflective band extending between the medial epicondyle (Med Ep) and sublime tubercle of the ulna (*arrows*).

separation of the torn ligament ends. Fluid can frequently be identified passing through the ligament from the joint into the adjacent soft tissues. Partial tears of the UCL are diagnosed when there is some preservation of ligamentous structure. In addition to the static ultrasound examination, the ligaments can also be scrutinized while applying an abduction force to the elbow, which may show dynamic instability.

Injury to the UCL can occur either directly from an acute valgus stress injury or elbow dislocation, or secondary to repetitive valgus overload in a throwing athlete. Most injuries involve the mid portion of the anterior bundle of the UCL, although proximal and distal avulsions can also occur.[16–18] In low-grade sprains the ligament fibers appear grossly intact but there is periligamentous edema (**Fig. 7**). In more significant injuries there is partial or complete disruption of ligament fibers (**Figs. 8 and 9**), often with concomitant injury to the adjacent flexor-pronator muscle group or ulnar nerve. In a study of baseball pitchers, MRI had a reported sensitivity and specificity of 100% for diagnosis of complete UCL tears, but only 14% sensitivity and 100% specificity for diagnosis of partial tears.[2] These figures may reflect subtle undersurface partial tears that can occur distally in athletes who throw, which characteristically spare the superficial fibers of the anterior bundle.[2,19] These partial tears can be difficult to detect on conventional MRI if no joint fluid is present, and MR arthrography may be necessary for diagnosis. Partial undersurface tears are characterized by distal extension of fluid or contrast along the medial margin of the coronoid process, forming the so-called T sign (**Fig. 10**).

Valgus stress injuries produce concurrent impaction forces in the lateral joint, which may result in osteochondral injuries of the radiocapitellar joint. Osteochondral injuries are best evaluated on MR arthrography, which allows visualization of articular cartilage defects and detection of small joint bodies, in addition to showing bone contusions.

Injuries of the UCL are commonly encountered in athletes participating in sports requiring an overhead throwing motion, such as volleyball, tennis, javelin, and baseball pitching. These sporting activities all require rapid forceful extension of the elbow,

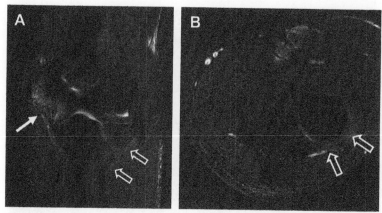

Fig. 7. (*A*) Coronal and (*B*) axial T2-weighted images with fat saturation showing mild edema around the anterior bundle of the UCL (*arrow*), although the fibers appear grossly intact. Reactive bone marrow edema is seen within the adjacent medial epicondyle and medial trochlea. Edema is also seen around the lateral ulnar collateral ligament (LUCL) as it passes behind the radial neck, compatible with a sprain (*open arrow*).

together with valgus stress and pronation of the supinated forearm. Maximal valgus stress is applied to the elbow in the late cocking and acceleration stages of throwing.[11] This movement combined with the rapid extension of the elbow can result in posteromedial shear forces. This repetitive microtrauma may eventually lead to posteromedial osteoarthritis, joint bodies, or olecranon stress fractures (**Fig. 11**).[11,20–23] This constellation of findings in athletes who throw constitutes valgus extension overload syndrome. On MRI the UCL can appear either thickened or attenuated in these athletes, and there may also be heterotopic ossification or hypertrophic bony spurring at the ulnar insertion (**Fig. 12**).

In skeletally immature individuals valgus extension overload leads to Little League elbow, characterized by medial epicondylar apophysitis. This condition manifests as

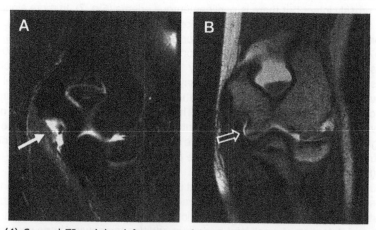

Fig. 8. (*A*) Coronal T2-weighted fat-saturated image shows a complete tear of the UCL (*arrow*), with edema in the adjacent flexor-pronator mass, suggesting an associated strain. (*B*) Coronal T1-weighted MR arthrographic image following ligamentous reconstruction in the same patient shows intact graft fibers (*open arrow*).

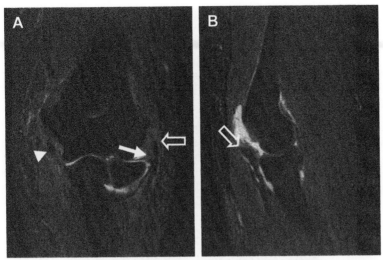

Fig. 9. (*A*) Coronal and (*B*) sagittal fat-saturated T2-weighted images after posterior elbow dislocation show a complete tear of the LUCL proximally (*arrow*), with avulsion of the common flexor tendon (*open arrow*). There is an associated moderate grade sprain of the UCL (*arrowhead*). The radial head is subluxed posteriorly with respect to the capitellum, consistent with PLRI.

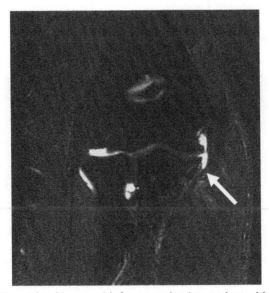

Fig. 10. Coronal T2-weighted image with fat saturation in a patient with a small joint effusion shows a partial undersurface tear of the distal UCL, with extension of fluid along the medial margin of the coronoid process (*arrow*).

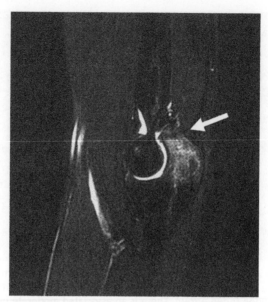

Fig. 11. Sagittal fat-saturated T2-weighted image in a 15-year-old baseball pitcher shows a stress fracture through the olecranon tip (*arrow*) with extensive bone marrow edema in the olecranon. (*Courtesy of* John MacKenzie, MD.)

fragmentation or distraction of the medial epicondylar apophysis on imaging, with corresponding high T2 signal intensity on MRI (**Fig. 13**).[24] Compressive forces in the lateral compartment can produce osteochondritis dissecans of the capitellum or radial head.[25,26]

Lateral Collateral Ligament Complex

The lateral collateral ligament complex has 3 main components: the radial collateral ligament proper (RCL), lateral UCL, and annular ligament. The RCL arises from the

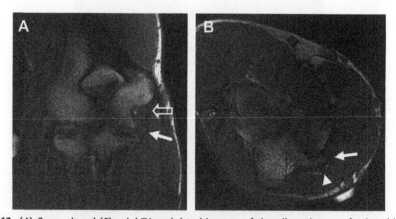

Fig. 12. (*A*) Coronal and (*B*) axial T1-weighted images of the elbow in a professional baseball pitcher show a thickened UCL (*open arrow*). A prominent bony spur is seen arising from the medial aspect of the coronoid process (*arrows*), and lying immediately adjacent to the ulnar nerve (*arrowhead*).

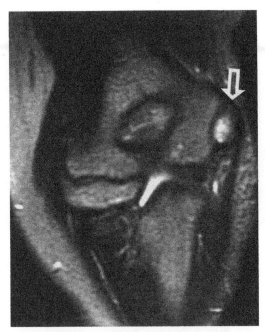

Fig. 13. Coronal T2-weighted image in a young pitcher showing bone marrow edema around the medial apophysis (*open arrow*) compatible with Little League elbow. (*Courtesy of* John D. MacKenzie, MD.)

lateral humeral epicondyle just deep to the common extensor tendon, and blends with fibers of the annular ligament, which surrounds the radial head. The LUCL arises from the lateral humeral condyle and passes behind the radial head to insert into the supinator crest of the ulna. The LUCL provides the primary restraint to varus stress at the elbow. On MRI the RCL and LUCL can be difficult to distinguish as separate structures, but are best visualized on sequential coronal images (**Fig. 14**), whereas the annular ligament is optimally visualized on axial images.

On ultrasound, the RCL is identified deep to the common extensor origin (**Fig. 15**). The meniscal homolog is a tiny fibrocartilage structure similar to that found adjacent to the triangular fibrocartilage complex in the wrist, sometimes referred to as the lateral plica. The meniscal homolog attaches to the RCL and helps to identify it. Disruption of the ligament shows similar characteristics to the UCL with the loss of the internal architecture.

The lateral collateral ligaments can be torn by an acute varus stress injury or elbow dislocation, which may result in posterolateral rotatory instability (PLRI) of the elbow.[27,28] The most common mechanism of injury is a fall on an outstretched hand with the forearm supinated. The resultant axial and valgus load tears the lateral collateral ligament complex, often leading to PLRI. Tears of the lateral collateral ligaments usually involve the humeral attachments, and are best depicted on coronal MR images.[24,29] Posterolateral subluxation of the radial head with respect to the capitellum can occur when the elbow is extended and the forearm is supinated. This condition is best seen on sagittal images (see **Fig. 9**).

LUCL disease can also be seen in patients with moderate to severe lateral epicondylitis (**Fig. 16**),[30,31] either as a direct result of degeneration and tearing in the adjacent

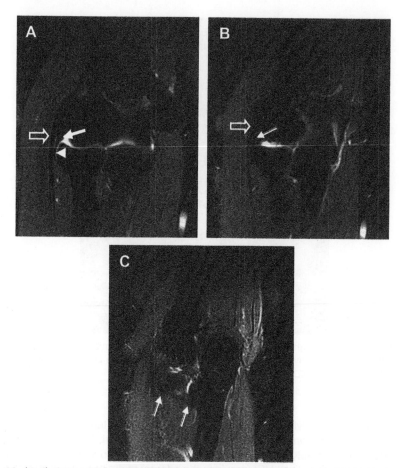

Fig. 14. (*A–C*) Sequential coronal fat-saturated T2-weighted images showing the RCL (*arrow*) lying deep to the common extensor tendon (*open arrow*) and blending with the annular ligament (*arrowhead*). On posterior images the LUCL (*small arrows*) can be seen passing behind the radial head to insert into the sublime tubercle of the ulna.

tendon, or potentially secondary to previous corticosteroid injections or overexuberant surgical debridement for common extensor tendon disease.

TENDON DISEASE
Lateral Tendon Disease

Lateral epicondylitis or tennis elbow is common in athletes involved in sports requiring overhead arm motions such as tennis, windsurfing, rock climbing, javelin throwing, and baseball pitching,[32] resulting in chronic symptoms and suboptimal athletic performance. This condition is believed to occur as a result of repetitive overloading of the extensor muscle mass, producing microtears with subsequent formation of granulation tissue or angiofibroblastic tendinosis.[29,33,34] Although areas of neovascularization can be seen on histology, inflammatory cells are not usually present, and this condition should perhaps more appropriately be called lateral epicondylosis or epicondylopathy. The extensor carpi radialis brevis tendon is usually the first component of the

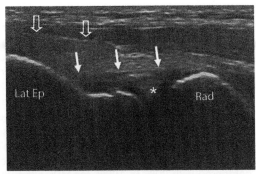

Fig. 15. Ultrasound image of the lateral elbow shows the radial collateral ligament (*arrows*) and meniscal homolog (*asterisk*), lying deep to the common extensor tendon (*open arrow*). Lat Ep, lateral epicondyle; Rad, radial head.

common extensor tendon to be affected, and there may be associated macroscopic tears. The diagnosis of lateral epicondylosis is usually made on clinical examination alone, and imaging is usually reserved for recalcitrant disease.

On MRI the common extensor tendon is seen as a low signal intensity band, just deep to the lateral collateral ligament complex (see **Fig. 14**). In lateral epicondylosis, the tendon usually appears thickened, with areas of increased T1 and T2 signal intensity corresponding to areas of angiofibroblastic tendinosis. Reactive edema may be seen within the surrounding soft tissues and lateral epicondyle. Fluid signal intensity may also be seen within the extensor carpi radialis brevis tendon, possibly signifying an underlying macroscopic tear,[29] although extensive edema without fiber disruption can be difficult to differentiate from partial tear on MRI. As mentioned earlier, the LUCL can be involved in patients with more severe disease, and should be carefully assessed in patients with lateral epicondylitis (see **Fig. 16**). If the tear of the LUCL is

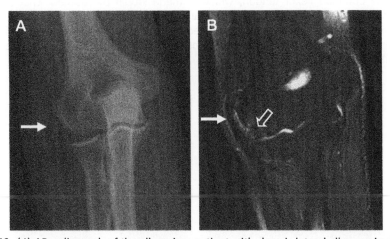

Fig. 16. (*A*) AP radiograph of the elbow in a patient with chronic lateral elbow pain shows focal soft tissue swelling over the lateral epicondyle, with mild underlying bony irregularity and a small focus of heterotopic calcification (*arrow*). (*B*) On the corresponding coronal T2-weighted image with fat saturation there is focal swelling and undersurface partial tearing of the common extensor tendon, with underlying bone marrow edema in the lateral epicondyle. There is also partial tearing of the proximal LUCL (*open arrow*).

not identified, surgical treatment addressing only the common extensor tendon may lead to further destabilization of the elbow and worsening symptoms.[35]

Sonography of the common extensor tendon can also be used to confirm a clinical diagnosis of lateral epicondylosis in patients with lateral elbow pain, and can also guide percutaneous therapy. Findings include swelling of the tendon, focal areas of decreased echogenicity, intratendinous calcification, focal fluid subjacent to the common extensor tendon in patients with a partial tear, and adjacent bone irregularity.[36–38] Less commonly reported in the literature but useful in the diagnosis is the presence of abnormal vessels that probably arise as a hypoxic response secondary to chronic injury, resulting in the production of vascular endothelial growth factor (**Fig. 17**). Studies have reported sensitivities of 64% to 88% for detection of epicondylitis by ultrasound, compared with 90% to 100% for MRI, although both modalities have similar specificity.[36,37] It is likely that improvements in ultrasound technology and the incorporation of abnormal Doppler signal increases the sensitivity of ultrasound. Use of ultrasound as a diagnostic tool has an additional advantage over MRI in that guided therapy can be applied immediately following diagnosis. Ultrasound-guided treatment includes dry needling of the tendon or injection of corticosteroid, autologous blood products, platelet-rich plasma, or other therapeutic agents.[39–43]

Medial Tendon Disease

Medial epicondylosis, commonly referred to as medial epicondylitis or golfer's elbow, is less common than its lateral counterpart, but often occurs in high-performance athletes, particularly in sports requiring repetitive valgus and flexion forces at the elbow such as golf, tennis, racquetball, baseball pitching, javelin, football, archery, and swimming.[20,44] Again this is believed to represent an overuse injury of the common flexor tendon caused by repetitive valgus overload, resulting in angiofibroblastic tendinosis and fibrillar degeneration of collagen.[45] Patients present with chronic medial elbow pain, exacerbated by activities requiring resisted flexion of wrist and pronation of the forearm. On physical examination, patients have point tenderness over the common flexor tendon, which is made worse by resisted wrist flexion. However, the clinical diagnosis of medial epicondylitis can be more challenging, because similar symptoms can be produced by UCL injuries, ulnar neuritis, or intraarticular disease.[20,44] Therefore, MRI can be helpful in the evaluation of patients presenting with medial elbow pain.

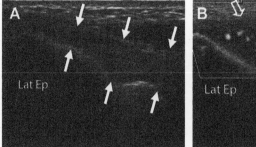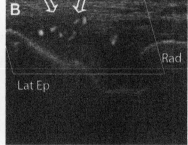

Fig. 17. (*A*) Coronal ultrasound image of a normal common extensor tendon arising from the lateral epicondyle (Lat Epi) and showing a parallel echogenic fibrillar pattern (*between arrows*). (*B*) Coronal ultrasound image in lateral epicondylitis shows focal swelling of the common extensor tendon, which appears hypoechoic with abnormal vasculature on color Doppler examination (*open arrows*).

The common flexor tendon is seen as a low signal intensity band arising from the medial humeral epicondyle on coronal images, just deep to the UCL and paralleling the long axis of the ulna (see **Fig. 6**). In medial epicondylosis, the common flexor tendon may appear thickened, with focal increased signal intensity within the tendon on both T1- and T2-weighted images (**Fig. 18**). Some patients develop macroscopic tears in the tendon, and reactive edema may be apparent in the surrounding soft tissues or medial epicondyle. Disease is most commonly localized to the flexor carpi radialis and pronator teres, which are the most anterior components of the common flexor origin. Larger tears may also involve the palmaris longus, flexor digitorum superficialis, and flexor carpi ulnaris. Patients with medial epicondylosis resulting from medial tension overload may show concurrent disease within the UCL or ulnar nerve.[46]

Ultrasound can also be used to evaluate the common flexor tendon, and guide percutaneous therapy in patients with medial epicondylosis. Focal hypoechoic areas can be seen within the common flexor tendon, and there may be accompanying tendon tears, intratendinous calcifications, or cortical irregularity,[47,48] indicating associated entheseal disease.

Anterior Tendon Disease

The biceps brachii muscle produces flexion of the elbow in conjunction with the brachialis, and is also a powerful supinator of the forearm. Distally the biceps tendon courses through the antecubital fossa to insert on to the bicipital tuberosity of the radius. However, some of the superficial tendon fibers sweep medially across the antecubital fossa to blend with the fascia of the flexor-pronator mass, forming the bicipital aponeurosis or lacertus fibrosis (**Fig. 19**). The distal biceps tendon comprises 2 components, one each from the long and short heads of the biceps brachii muscle. The short head component is more superficial and inserts more distally.

Rupture of the distal biceps tendon is an uncommon injury in athletes, but may be seen in weight lifters and body builders, particularly if they are smokers or are taking anabolic steroids.[49,50] Distal biceps rupture typically results from a sudden extension force applied to the arm with the elbow held in 90° of flexion, or from forceful

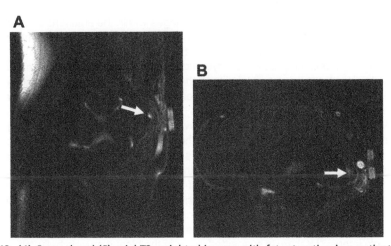

Fig. 18. (A) Coronal and (B) axial T2-weighted images with fat saturation in a patient with chronic medial elbow pain shows focal increased T2 signal within the common flexor tendon (*arrow*), with edema in the adjacent soft tissues. The patient was imaged with the arm at the side, producing poor fat saturation peripherally.

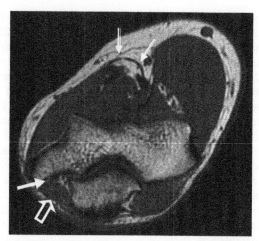

Fig. 19. Axial T1-weighted image showing an anconeus epitrochlearis muscle (*open arrow*) behind the medial epicondyle. There is loss of the normal cuff of fat around the ulnar nerve (*arrow*), although the nerve itself appears of normal caliber. An intact bicipital aponeurosis can be seen anteriorly (*double arrows*).

hyperextension against resistance. This situation may cause the biceps tendon to avulse from the bicipital tuberosity of the radius, and if the bicipital aponeurosis is also torn, the tendon end retracts into the upper arm, producing a palpable defect on physical examination. However, if the bicipital aponeurosis remains intact, there is only minimal retraction of the tendon, which can make differentiation from a partial tear difficult.[51] Several factors are believed to predispose to a distal biceps tendon tear, including tendon degeneration and the relative hypovascularity of the distal tendon, which limits repair mechanisms in this region.[51–53] Repetitive traction forces may produce bony hypertrophy of the bicipital tuberosity, which may cause mechanical impingement of the distal biceps when the forearm is pronated, leading to partial tendon tears. The distal biceps tendon also lacks a tendon sheath, and mechanical impingement can also cause inflammatory changes within the adjacent bicipitoradial bursae, which further aggravates the situation.[52,54] Partial tears also make the tendon more susceptible to rupture with insignificant trauma.

Tears of the biceps muscle belly or myotendinous strains are less common, but may occur following direct trauma.[55] Injuries to the brachialis muscle are uncommon, but may result from eccentric muscle contraction against resistance or posterior elbow dislocations.[56,57]

On MRI the distal biceps tendon is best evaluated on sagittal and axial images. In chronic disease, the biceps tendon may either appear thickened or attenuated with associated partial tears and cubital bursitis (**Fig. 20**).[54,58,59] In acute rupture, the tendon appears discontinuous distally, with surrounding edema and hemorrhage (**Fig. 21**). The tendon can retract proximally if the bicipital aponeurosis is torn. Usually the elbow is imaged in the extended position. However, in patients specifically suspected of distal biceps disease, the so-called FABS position (flexion, abduction, and supination) can be used, which facilitates visualization of the entire biceps tendon on a single image.[60] If there is suspected injury of the biceps muscle belly rather than the distal tendon, the field of view should be extended to cover the upper arm (**Fig. 22**).

Ultrasound can also be used to evaluate the distal biceps tendon, which shows parallel echogenic fibers, inserting into the bicipital tuberosity of the radius (**Fig. 23**).

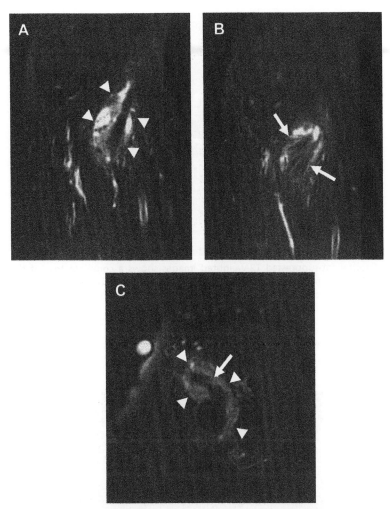

Fig. 20. (*A, B*) Sagittal and (*C*) axial fat-suppressed T2-weighted images show thickening of the distal biceps tendon, with a high-grade partial tear (*arrows*) and surrounding cubital bursitis (*arrowheads*).

Ultrasound can be used to detect tendinosis, tendon tears, and peritendinous fluid collections (see **Fig. 23**). Dynamic ultrasound in flexion and extension is helpful to differentiate between partial or complete tendon tears.[1,61–63] However, the oblique course of the tendon in the antecubital fossa can make visualization of the tendon insertion difficult in the longitudinal plane. The insertion can also be evaluated from a dorsal approach with the forearm pronated, which brings the bicipital tuberosity and tendon insertion into view.[52,64] A more recent paper has also described a lateral approach to evaluate the distal tendon,[65] with the arm held in the FABS position. However, we recommend an approach from the medial or ulnar side to allow a more complete assessment of the tendon insertion.

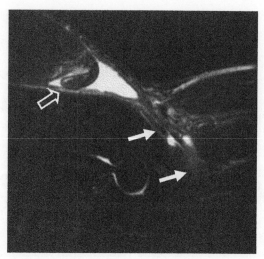

Fig. 21. Sagittal fat-suppressed T2-weighted images shows a complete tear of the distal biceps tendon with retraction of the tendon end (*open arrow*) surrounded by hematoma. Edema tracks toward the prior tendon insertion site into the bicipital tuberosity of the radius (*arrows*).

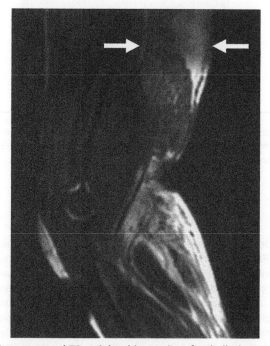

Fig. 22. Sagittal fat-suppressed T2-weighted image in a football player sustaining a direct blow to his upper arm. There is a high-grade rupture of the muscle belly (*arrows*), with extensive hemorrhage and edema tracking distally.

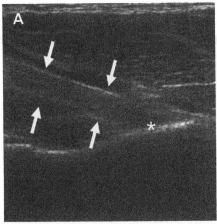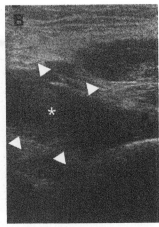

Fig. 23. Sagittal ultrasound of the upper arm in (*A*) normal tendon and (*B*) an athlete with avulsion of the distal biceps tendon. The normal tendon (*arrows*) can be followed to its distal end (*asterisk*) inserting into the radial tuberosity. (*B*) The biceps tendon is torn and its tip retracted (*asterisk*) and the empty sheath is fluid filled (*arrowheads*).

Posterior Tendon Disease

Rupture of the triceps tendon is uncommon, and typically occurs from a fall on an outstretched hand. This condition may be associated with fractures of the radial head, which are sustained via a similar mechanism of injury.[66,67] Less common mechanisms include a direct blow to the posterior elbow or forceful eccentric contraction of the triceps muscle with the elbow flexed, which may occur in athletes participating in high-impact sports such as football, rugby, or soccer.[68] The triceps tendon can also rupture in weight lifters from severe sustained contraction, particularly if the patient is taking anabolic steroids and has coexistent tendinosis.[69,70] Additional risk factors include oral or injected corticosteroids, olecranon bursitis, inflammatory arthritis, or renal insufficiency with hyperparathyroidism.[51,71–73] Partial tears of the triceps tendon, rupture of the muscle belly, or myotendinous strains are rare.[71,74–76]

The triceps tendon usually avulses from the olecranon process, and a palpable defect can be detected on physical examination. Radiographs should be obtained in cases of suspected triceps tendon ruptures to look for a small flake fracture of the olecranon or a radial head fracture. Both MRI and ultrasound can be used to confirm the diagnosis, and are helpful in differentiating between partial and complete tears. MRI shows a gap within the distal triceps tendon in complete tears, and can be used to assess the degree of retraction of the tendon end. Hemorrhage and edema are often seen within the surrounding soft tissue and olecranon bursa (**Fig. 24**). Occasionally complete and partial rupture can be difficult to differentiate if the tendon ends are overlapping. In these cases, dynamic ultrasound clarifies the diagnosis.[1] In more chronic disease, degenerative changes may be seen within the tendon, similar to that seen in the biceps tendon, with partial ruptures showing interruption of tendon fibers and focal fluid (**Fig. 25**).

Sonographic evaluation of the posterior elbow can be used to evaluate the triceps tendon (**Fig. 26**), but is also helpful in the diagnosis and treatment of olecranon bursitis, as well as posterior joint effusion and detection of joint bodies.

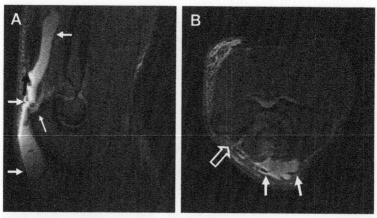

Fig. 24. Sagittal (*A*) and axial (*B*) fat-suppressed T2-weighted images in a 22-year-old jiu jitsu fighter shows avulsion of the triceps tendon (*black arrow*), with extensive hemorrhage in the olecranon bursa (*arrows*). A possible small cortical defect is seen at the olecranon (*long arrow*), although this was not apparent radiographically. Edema is seen extending around the ulnar nerve (*open arrow*), accounting for why patients may also complain of ulnar nerve symptoms.

NEURAL INJURIES

Nerve disease around the elbow is common, as the main nerves are located in a superficial position, and are in close proximity to underlying osseous structures, making them vulnerable to acute injury from a direct blow or underlying fracture. Nerves also pass through narrow fibromuscular or fibro-osseous tunnels around the elbow, where they can be compressed, resulting in entrapment neuropathy. Nerves pass directly through muscles that are extremely active during throwing, making athletes who throw prone to dynamic compression syndromes.[77]

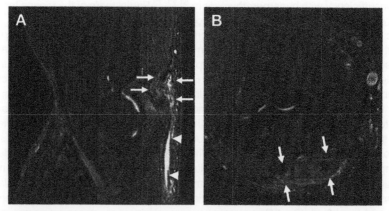

Fig. 25. Sagittal (*A*) and axial (*B*) fat-suppressed T2-weighted images in a patient with partial tearing of the distal triceps tendon. There is thickening and irregularity of the distal tendon (*arrows*) with peritendinous edema and fluid in the olecranon bursa (*arrowheads*), and reactive bone marrow edema is seen within the olecranon process.

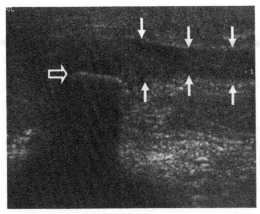

Fig. 26. Sagittal ultrasound of the posterior elbow showing an avulsion fracture from the olecranon (*open arrow*), with the triceps tendon inserting into the bony fragment (*arrows*). Echogenic fat is seen within the olecranon fossa.

Symptoms of nerve compression include sensory changes such as burning pain, numbness, and paresthesia, and motor weakness, which can be debilitating in athletes who throw. The diagnosis is usually confirmed by electromyography or nerve conduction studies. However, imaging is helpful because it can both confirm the diagnosis and identify any neural compressive lesions or anatomic variants that may help localize the site of compression.[46,78,79] Normal nerves appear of intermediate to low signal intensity on all pulse sequences. Compressed or entrapped nerves may show an abrupt change in caliber as well as increased T2 signal intensity proximal or distal to the compression site. MRI can also show the secondary changes of denervation in affected muscles, such as hypertrophy and edema, which can appear within 24 to 48 hours of denervation. In chronic denervation muscle, atrophy and fatty infiltration can be seen within the affected muscles. More recently high-resolution ultrasound has also become an effective and low-cost alternative to MRI for showing compression and entrapment neuropathies.[80–83]

Nerves have a distinct appearance on ultrasound. The neural bundles themselves appear dark against a background of bright perineural matrix. This image can resemble the appearance of tendons; however, the nerve fibers are generally larger and more continuous than their tendinous counterparts. A clinical advantage of ultrasound is that the nerve can be traced throughout its entire length; for example, the median nerve can be followed from the brachial plexus through the arm, elbow, forearm, and carpal tunnel. Such extensive coverage is possible with MRI but is more time consuming. Sonopalpation can also be used to elicit the equivalent of a clinical Tinel sign, which can help to localize the area of nerve compression. Ultrasound is most frequently used to detect changes in nerve morphology at the level of compression. Secondary signs include alterations in echotexture, constrained movement, and, occasionally, changes in perineural vascularity. If an artery accompanies a particular nerve through its fibro-osseous tunnel, changes in flow characteristics compared with the contralateral side may be detected. Examining the elbow in different positions may cause pressure changes to augment these findings.

Ulnar Nerve

Ulnar nerve compression is the most frequently seen peripheral neuropathy around the elbow, and commonly occurs in athletes who throw. The ulnar nerve is under increased tension during the throwing motion, and the pressure within the cubital tunnel has been shown to increase with flexion, making the ulnar nerve particularly susceptible to compression during the late cocking phase of throwing.[77] Trauma to the UCL or valgus extension overload, particularly where osteophytes have formed, can also result in ulnar neuritis. Ulnar nerve disease may present with aching pain and discomfort over the medial elbow and forearm. Transient numbness and paresthesia can occur over the medial aspect of the forearm and hand. Athletes may complain of clumsiness or heaviness in their throwing arm, with easy fatigue and loss of throwing speed.

There are several potential sites of compression, but the most common is in the cubital tunnel, a tight fibro-osseous tunnel on the posterior aspect of the medial epicondyle and medial olecranon. The floor of the cubital tunnel is formed by the joint capsule and posterior bundle of the UCL. The roof is formed by the cubital tunnel retinaculum (Osborne ligament) proximally and the aponeurosis of the flexor carpi ulnaris (arcuate ligament) distally. The space within the cubital tunnel naturally decreases with elbow flexion as the aponeurosis of the flexor carpi ulnaris becomes taut, which can be problematic in athletes who throw. Several anatomic variants can predispose an individual to developing ulnar neuritis. These variants include thickening of the cubital tunnel retinaculum, seen in 22% of the population, and a small anomalous muscle called the anconeus epitrochlearis that traverses the cubital tunnel, seen in up to 23% of the population (see **Fig. 19**). In 10% of the population, the cubital tunnel retinaculum is completely absent. This situation allows the ulnar nerve to sublux anteriorly over the medial epicondyle during flexion, which may lead to friction neuritis.[84–87] Although this condition can be present in the normal population, a repeated throwing motion in an athlete may lead to repetitive microtrauma of the ulnar nerve. Ultrasound can be helpful to evaluate for ulnar nerve subluxation dynamically.

There are several other potential sites for ulnar nerve entrapment in an athlete who throws including a hypertrophied medial head of the triceps muscle,[87–89] the arcade of Struthers, which is a thick fascial band running between the intermuscular septum and medial triceps,[90,91] fascial bands between the 2 heads of the flexor carpi ulnaris,[92] and the deep flexor-pronator aponeurosis.[93]

On MRI, the ulnar nerve is best seen on axial MR images, and is normally located within the cubital tunnel posterior to the medial humeral epicondyle, surrounded by a cuff of fat. In ulnar neuritis, the ulnar nerve can appear flattened at the site of obstruction, with obliteration of the surrounding fat. There is often focal or diffuse swelling of the ulnar nerve, with increased signal intensity on T2-weighted or inversion recovery sequences (**Fig. 27**). Ultrasound can also show changes in caliber of the ulnar nerve at the level of the cubital tunnel (**Fig. 28**), but has the advantage of dynamic evaluation for ulnar nerve subluxation (**Fig. 29**). The ulnar nerve may be deviated from its normal position by a space-occupying lesion, scarring, posteromedial arthritis, or synovitis, which can be detected on both MRI and ultrasound.

Median Nerve

Median nerve entrapment is less common than ulnar nerve disease, but again can occur in athletes who throw. Compression of the median nerve around the elbow can present in 2 clinically distinct ways. Pronator syndrome is the most common, presenting with pain over the volar aspect of the forearm, and numbness and paresthesia in the median nerve distribution. Symptoms are worsened with repetitive rotatory movements of the forearm, or repetitive extension and pronation in athletes who throw.[77] In anterior interosseous syndrome or Kiloh-Nevin syndrome, there is selective compression of a motor branch, resulting in weakness of the flexor pollicis longus,

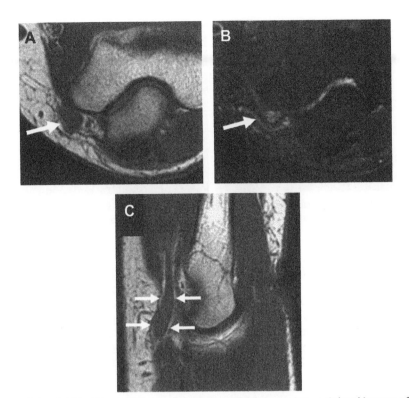

Fig. 27. (*A*) Axial T1-, (*B*) axial fat-suppressed T2-, and (*C*) coronal T1-weighted images of the elbow in a patient with ulnar neuritis and absence of the cubital tunnel retinaculum. There is focal swelling of the ulnar nerve (*arrows*), which resembles a green onion or cobra shape on the coronal image.

flexor digitorum profundus to the second and third digits, and the pronator quadratus muscle. Although this condition is uncommon in athletes, it can occur in throwers as a result of cumulative injury, violent muscle contraction, or even overaggressive exercises of the forearm.[77]

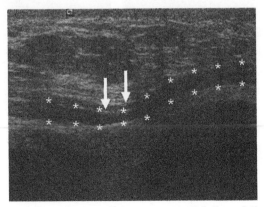

Fig. 28. Longitudinal ultrasound image of the posteromedial elbow following the course of the ulnar nerve (*asterisks*) in an athlete with ulnar neuritis. There is focal compression of the ulnar nerve at the level of the cubital tunnel (*arrows*).

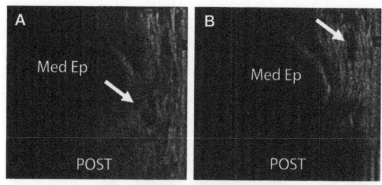

Fig. 29. Transverse ultrasound images of the medial elbow in (*A*) extension and (*B*) flexion showing anterior subluxation of the ulnar nerve over the medial epicondyle (Med Ep) during flexion (*arrow*).

Compression of the median nerve usually occurs at one of 4 potential sites: the supracondylar process and ligament of Struthers, the bicipital aponeurosis, the pronator teres muscle, and the proximal arch of the flexor digitorum superficialis muscle. The supracondylar process is a small bony spur projecting from the anterior aspect of the distal humerus, which can be identified on lateral radiographs (**Fig. 30**). The ligament of Struthers is a fibrous band extending from the supracondylar spur to the medial epicondyle, which forms a fibro-osseous tunnel that may entrap the median

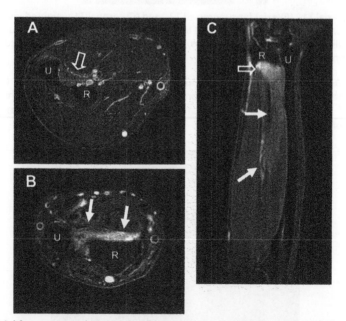

Fig. 30. Axial fat-suppressed T2-weighted images through the (*A*) mid and (*B*) distal forearm show edema within the flexor digitorum profundus (FDP) muscle supplying the index and middle fingers (*open arrow*) and the pronator quadratus muscle (PQ) (*open arrow*), compatible with anterior interosseous nerve syndrome. (*C*) The edema can be seen extending into the mid forearm on the coronal fat-saturated T2-weighted image. R, radius; U, ulna.

nerve and occasionally the brachial artery.[94–96] The median nerve then enters the antecubital fossa, and lies medial to the biceps tendon and brachial artery, where it may be compressed by a thickened bicipital aponeurosis or an accessory fibrous band associated with an anomalous third head of the biceps muscle.[97] However, the most common site of compression is where the median nerve leaves the antecubital fossa by passing between the superficial and deep heads of the pronator teres muscle, where fibrous bands can occur. These bands can cause selective compression of the anterior interosseous branch, just as it diverges from the median nerve. In athletes who throw, the pronator teres muscle may be hypertrophied, resulting in compression or irritation of the median nerve with repetitive pronation and extension of the elbow.[77] The most distal site of compression occurs at the proximal margin of the flexor digitorum superficialis, where a fibrous band can occur.[59,98] Other causes of compression include elbow dislocation or fracture, anomalous muscles such as an accessory head of the flexor pollicis longus (Gantzer muscle), anomalous vessels, vascular disease, or a distended bicipitoradial bursa.[99–101]

A patient presenting with symptoms suggesting median nerve compression should initially have radiographs to exclude a supracondylar spur (**Fig. 31**). On MRI, the median nerve is not so well visualized as the ulnar nerve around the elbow because of a paucity of perineural fat, making it difficult to visualize morphologic changes within the nerve. However, MRI may detect space-occupying lesions or accessory muscles, and can visualize the secondary signs of nerve compression, namely edema and atrophy, in affected forearm musculature (see **Fig. 30**).[102]

Radial Nerve

Radial nerve injury around the elbow is uncommon, and as symptoms are nonspecific, the diagnosis is often delayed. Compression of the radial nerve at the elbow can present as either radial tunnel syndrome or posterior interosseous syndrome. The radial tunnel is the most common site of compression, and begins at the level of the

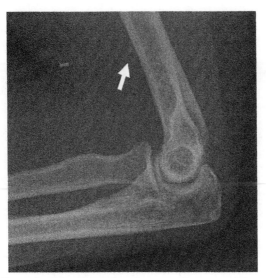

Fig. 31. Lateral radiograph of the elbow showing a small supracondylar spur (*arrow*) arising from the anterior aspect of the distal humerus.

radiocapitellar joint, extending to the distal margin of the supinator muscle. The radial nerve divides into superficial and deep branches at the proximal border of the supinator muscle. The deep branch or posterior interosseous nerve is a motor nerve, innervating the supinator and most of the wrist and finger extensors. Selective compression of the posterior interosseous nerve produces a motor palsy, leading to weakness of the wrist and hand extensors. The superficial branch of the radial nerve is sensory, supplying sensation to the dorsal and lateral aspects of the wrist and hand. Radial tunnel syndrome is characterized as pain along the lateral elbow and forearm, which can mimic lateral epicondylitis.[77] However, an accurate diagnosis may be difficult, as both conditions can present with similar symptoms, and radial tunnel syndrome can occur in conjunction with lateral epicondylitis.

The radial nerve can be compressed proximal to the antecubital fossa by a fibrous arch in the lateral head of the triceps muscle. Entrapment in this location may occur after strenuous muscular effort, leading to weakness of forearm supination and wrist extension.[103,104] Both radial tunnel syndrome and posterior interosseous nerve syndrome occur from identical sites of compression at the elbow. The nerve may be compressed by fibrous bands around the radiocapitellar joint, the tendinous edge of the extensor carpi radialis brevis, or vascular arcades of the recurrent radial artery, known as the leash of Henry. The 2 most common sites of radial nerve compression are at the arcade of Frohse, a fibrous arch occurring within the superficial head of the supinator, or fibrous bands occurring within the distal supinator.[77,98] Compression of the radial nerve or posterior interosseous nerve can also result from trauma, space-occupying lesions, or inflammatory change.[105]

Both radial tunnel syndrome and posterior interosseous nerve syndrome have similar appearances on MRI. MRI may show the cause of nerve compression, such as inflamed bursae, ganglia, thickening of the leading age of the extensor carpi radialis brevis, or prominent radial recurrent arcades.[105] Edema and fatty infiltration or atrophy can occur within the supinator muscle and extensor muscles of the forearm (**Fig. 32**).

BONE AND CARTILAGE INJURY

Within the elbow joint, injury to the articular surface is most commonly encountered on the radial aspect of the joint, where the convex surface of the capitellum is most

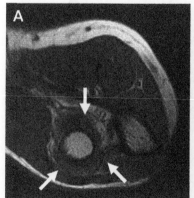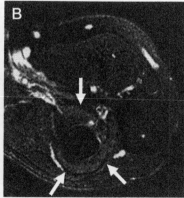

Fig. 32. (*A*) Axial T1- and (*B*) T2-weighted images through the proximal forearm in a patient with symptoms suggesting posterior interosseous syndrome show mild atrophy and edema within the supinator muscle (*arrows*).

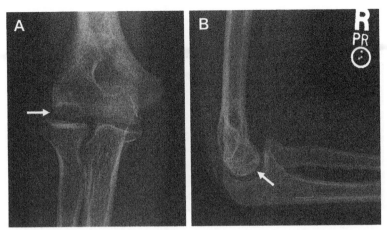

Fig. 33. (A) AP and (B) lateral views of the elbow in a former gymnast showing flattening and lucency within the capitellum, compatible with osteochondritis dissecans.

vulnerable. Chronic compression injury is often seen in young athletes involved in sports placing repetitive valgus stress on the elbow, such as gymnasts and adolescent pitchers.[106] Plain radiographs are often normal in early disease, but may subsequently show flattening, subchondral sclerosis, and lysis located in the anteroinferior aspect of the capitellum (**Fig. 33**). In the acute phase, a joint effusion is often present. Bony abnormalities detected in young patients less than the age of 12 years are often self-limiting, and this condition is sometimes referred to as Panner disease. In older patients, cartilage disease may progress to a full thickness lesion. In later stages, a crack may form between the subchondral plate and underlying bone, leading to an osteochondral fragment that is loose in situ. Ultimately, separation may occur and a loose body is formed.

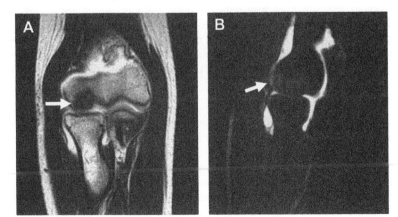

Fig. 34. (A) Coronal T1-weighted image in an adolescent tennis player shows focal low T1 signal within the capitellum (*arrow*). (B) The corresponding sagittal fat-saturated T2-weighted image shows bony irregularity of the anterior capitellum, with associated bone marrow edema compatible with osteochondritis dissecans. The overlying articular cartilage appears grossly intact.

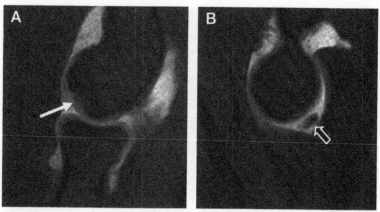

Fig. 35. Two sagittal fat-saturated T2-weighted images of the elbow following MR arthrography showing (*A*) a focal osteochondral defect of the capitellum (*arrow*). (*B*) A corresponding joint body is identified within the trochlear notch (*open arrow*).

MRI is used to more accurately depict the state of the articular cartilage, and its sensitivity is increased by the addition of intraarticular contrast. MRI can provide useful information on the size, location, and stability of the lesion (**Fig. 34**). Unstable lesions are usually larger, and are characterized by fluid tracking around the osteochondral lesion, or underlying cystic change.[106] MR arthrography can also determine the location of any detached intraarticular bodies (**Fig. 35**). Patients in whom MRI is contraindicated may benefit from CT arthography.

One potential pitfall in the diagnosis of osteochondral injury is the pseudodefect of the capitellum. The convex articular surface of the capitellum is directed anteriorly, and there is an abrupt transition between the posterior aspect of the articular surface and adjacent nonarticular surface of the lateral humeral condyle. A coronal slice through this transition point can simulate an underlying osteochondral lesion, and care should be taken not to misinterpret a pseudodefect of the capitellum as significant disease. The pseudodefect of the capitellum is inferoposterior in location, and has smoother margins than true osteochondral defects, which are usually found anteroinferiorly.

As most osteochondral injuries in young patients are anteroinferiorly located, many can be seen using ultrasound.[107] This characteristic can be particularly useful in very young patients, who may be frightened of undergoing an MRI examination.

SUMMARY

Elbow pain is a common complaint in athletes, usually occurring as a result of direct trauma or overuse. Standard radiographs are recommended if the patient has sustained acute injury, and may also provide useful information in athletes with chronic symptoms. However, MRI is the imaging modality of choice for the investigation of patients with both acute and chronic elbow pathologic conditions. Ultrasound can also be used to interrogate superficial anatomic structures, and has the advantage of dynamic evaluation and color Doppler examination. Portable ultrasound machines are now available, which may allow evaluation of the athlete immediately after sustaining acute injury. Although many sports injuries can be diagnosed from the clinical history and physical examination alone, medical imaging can be used to confirm the diagnosis, evaluate the extent of disease, and guide subsequent treatment.

REFERENCES

1. Kijowski R, De Smet AA. The role of ultrasound in the evaluation of sports medicine injuries of the upper extremity. Clin Sports Med 2006;25(3):569–90, viii.
2. Timmerman LA, Schwartz ML, Andrews JR. Preoperative evaluation of the ulnar collateral ligament by magnetic resonance imaging and computed tomography arthrography. Evaluation in 25 baseball players with surgical confirmation. Am J Sports Med 1994;22(1):26–31 [discussion: 32].
3. Dubberley JH, Faber KJ, Patterson SD, et al. The detection of loose bodies in the elbow: the value of MRI and CT arthrography. J Bone Joint Surg Br 2005; 87(5):684–6.
4. Waldt S, Bruegel M, Ganter K, et al. Comparison of multislice CT arthrography and MR arthrography for the detection of articular cartilage lesions of the elbow. Eur Radiol 2005;15(4):784–91.
5. Steinbach LS, Palmer WE, Schweitzer ME. Special focus session. MR arthrography. Radiographics 2002;22(5):1223–46.
6. Tuite MJ, Kijowski R. Sports-related injuries of the elbow: an approach to MRI interpretation. Clin Sports Med 2006;25(3):387–408, v.
7. Sinha AK, Kaeding CC, Wadley GM. Upper extremity stress fractures in athletes: clinical features of 44 cases. Clin J Sport Med 1999;9(4):199–202.
8. Van der Wall H, Frater CJ, Magee MA, et al. A novel view for the scintigraphic assessment of the elbow. Nucl Med Commun 1999;20(11):1059–65.
9. Pienimaki TT, Takalo RJ, Ahonen AK, et al. Three-phase bone scintigraphy in chronic epicondylitis. Arch Phys Med Rehabil 2008;89(11):2180–4.
10. Alcid JG, Ahmad CS, Lee TQ. Elbow anatomy and structural biomechanics. Clin Sports Med 2004;23(4):503–17, vii.
11. Lynch JR, Waitayawinyu T, Hanel DP, et al. Medial collateral ligament injury in the overhand-throwing athlete. J Hand Surg Am 2008;33(3):430–7.
12. Fowler KA, Chung CB. Normal MR imaging anatomy of the elbow. Magn Reson Imaging Clin N Am 2004;12(2):191–206, v.
13. Schwartz ML, al-Zahrani S, Morwessel RM, et al. Ulnar collateral ligament injury in the throwing athlete: evaluation with saline-enhanced MR arthrography. Radiology 1995;197(1):297–9.
14. Munshi M, Pretterklieber ML, Chung CB, et al. Anterior bundle of ulnar collateral ligament: evaluation of anatomic relationships by using MR imaging, MR arthrography, and gross anatomic and histologic analysis. Radiology 2004;231 (3):797–803.
15. Fowler KA, Chung CB. Normal MR imaging anatomy of the elbow. Radiol Clin North Am 2006;44(4):553–67, viii.
16. Salvo JP, Rizio L 3rd, Zvijac JE, et al. Avulsion fracture of the ulnar sublime tubercle in overhead throwing athletes. Am J Sports Med 2002;30(3):426–31.
17. Conway JE, Jobe FW, Glousman RE, et al. Medial instability of the elbow in throwing athletes. Treatment by repair or reconstruction of the ulnar collateral ligament. J Bone Joint Surg Am 1992;74(1):67–83.
18. Azar FM, Andrews JR, Wilk KE, et al. Operative treatment of ulnar collateral ligament injuries of the elbow in athletes. Am J Sports Med 2000;28(1):16–23.
19. Timmerman LA, Andrews JR. Undersurface tear of the ulnar collateral ligament in baseball players. A newly recognized lesion. Am J Sports Med 1994;22(1):33–6.
20. Chen FS, Rokito AS, Jobe FW. Medial elbow problems in the overhead-throwing athlete. J Am Acad Orthop Surg 2001;9(2):99–113.

21. Safran MR. Ulnar collateral ligament injury in the overhead athlete: diagnosis and treatment. Clin Sports Med 2004;23(4):643–63, x.
22. Ahmad CS, ElAttrache NS. Valgus extension overload syndrome and stress injury of the olecranon. Clin Sports Med 2004;23(4):665–76, x.
23. Schickendantz MS, Ho CP, Koh J. Stress injury of the proximal ulna in professional baseball players. Am J Sports Med 2002;30(5):737–41.
24. Kaplan LJ, Potter HG. MR imaging of ligament injuries to the elbow. Radiol Clin North Am 2006;44(4):583–94, ix.
25. Klingele KE, Kocher MS. Little league elbow: valgus overload injury in the paediatric athlete. Sports Med 2002;32(15):1005–15.
26. Ouellette H, Bredella M, Labis J, et al. MR imaging of the elbow in baseball pitchers. Skeletal Radiol 2008;37(2):115–21.
27. Charalambous CP, Stanley JK. Posterolateral rotatory instability of the elbow. J Bone Joint Surg Br 2008;90(3):272–9.
28. Singleton SB, Conway JE. PLRI: posterolateral rotatory instability of the elbow. Clin Sports Med 2004;23(4):629–42, ix–x.
29. Potter HG, Hannafin JA, Morwessel RM, et al. Lateral epicondylitis: correlation of MR imaging, surgical, and histopathologic findings. Radiology 1995;196(1):43–6.
30. Bredella MA, Tirman PF, Fritz RC, et al. MR imaging findings of lateral ulnar collateral ligament abnormalities in patients with lateral epicondylitis. AJR Am J Roentgenol 1999;173(5):1379–82.
31. Kalainov DM, Cohen MS. Posterolateral rotatory instability of the elbow in association with lateral epicondylitis. A report of three cases. J Bone Joint Surg Am 2005;87(5):1120–5.
32. Hume PA, Reid D, Edwards T. Epicondylar injury in sport: epidemiology, type, mechanisms, assessment, management and prevention. Sports Med 2006; 36(2):151–70.
33. Nirschl RP, Ashman ES. Elbow tendinopathy: tennis elbow. Clin Sports Med 2003;22(4):813–36.
34. Whaley AL, Baker CL. Lateral epicondylitis. Clin Sports Med 2004;23(4):677–91, x.
35. Morrey BE. Surgical failure of the tennis elbow. In: Morrey BF, editor. The elbow and its disorders. Philadelphia: Saunders; 1993. p. 553–9.
36. Levin D, Nazarian LN, Miller TT, et al. Lateral epicondylitis of the elbow: US findings. Radiology 2005;237(1):230–4.
37. Miller TT, Shapiro MA, Schultz E, et al. Comparison of sonography and MRI for diagnosing epicondylitis. J Clin Ultrasound 2002;30(4):193–202.
38. Connell D, Burke F, Coombes P, et al. Sonographic examination of lateral epicondylitis. AJR Am J Roentgenol 2001;176(3):777–82.
39. Zhu J, Hu B, Xing C, et al. Ultrasound-guided, minimally invasive, percutaneous needle puncture treatment for tennis elbow. Adv Ther 2008;25(10):1031–6.
40. Torp-Pedersen TE, Torp-Pedersen ST, Qvistgaard E, et al. Effect of glucocorticosteroid injections in tennis elbow verified on colour Doppler ultrasonography: evidence of inflammation. Br J Sports Med 2008;42(12):978–82.
41. Connell DA, Ali KE, Ahmad M, et al. Ultrasound-guided autologous blood injection for tennis elbow. Skeletal Radiol 2006;35(6):371–7.
42. Calfee RP, Patel A, DaSilva MF, et al. Management of lateral epicondylitis: current concepts. J Am Acad Orthop Surg 2008;16(1):19–29.
43. Faro F, Wolf JM. Lateral epicondylitis: review and current concepts. J Hand Surg Am 2007;32(8):1271–9.
44. Ciccotti MC, Schwartz MA, Ciccotti MG. Diagnosis and treatment of medial epicondylitis of the elbow. Clin Sports Med 2004;23(4):693–705, xi.

45. Ollivierre CO, Nirschl RP, Pettrone FA. Resection and repair for medial tennis elbow. A prospective analysis. Am J Sports Med 1995;23(2):214–21.
46. Kijowski R, De Smet AA. Magnetic resonance imaging findings in patients with medial epicondylitis. Skeletal Radiol 2005;34(4):196–202.
47. Park GY, Lee SM, Lee MY. Diagnostic value of ultrasonography for clinical medial epicondylitis. Arch Phys Med Rehabil 2008;89(4):738–42.
48. Suresh SP, Ali KE, Jones H, et al. Medial epicondylitis: is ultrasound guided autologous blood injection an effective treatment? Br J Sports Med 2006; 40(11):935–9 [discussion: 939].
49. Safran MR, Graham SM. Distal biceps tendon ruptures: incidence, demographics, and the effect of smoking. Clin Orthop Relat Res 2002;404:275–83.
50. Visuri T, Lindholm H. Bilateral distal biceps tendon avulsions with use of anabolic steroids. Med Sci Sports Exerc 1994;26(8):941–4.
51. Vidal AF, Drakos MC, Allen AA. Biceps tendon and triceps tendon injuries. Clin Sports Med 2004;23(4):707–22, xi.
52. Chew ML, Giuffre BM. Disorders of the distal biceps brachii tendon. Radiographics 2005;25(5):1227–37.
53. Seiler JG 3rd, Parker LM, Chamberland PD, et al. The distal biceps tendon. Two potential mechanisms involved in its rupture: arterial supply and mechanical impingement. J Shoulder Elbow Surg 1995;4(3):149–56.
54. Williams BD, Schweitzer ME, Weishaupt D, et al. Partial tears of the distal biceps tendon: MR appearance and associated clinical findings. Skeletal Radiol 2001; 30(10):560–4.
55. Schamblin ML, Safran MR. Injury of the distal biceps at the musculotendinous junction. J Shoulder Elbow Surg 2007;16(2):208–12.
56. Nishida Y, Tsukushi S, Yamada Y, et al. Brachialis muscle tear mimicking an intramuscular tumor: a report of two cases. J Hand Surg Am 2007;32(8):1237–41.
57. Van den Berghe GR, Queenan JF, Murphy DA. Isolated rupture of the brachialis: a case report. J Bone Joint Surg Am 2001;83(7):1074–5.
58. Durr HR, Stabler A, Pfahler M, et al. Partial rupture of the distal biceps tendon. Clin Orthop Relat Res 2000;374:195–200.
59. Kijowski R, Tuite M, Sanford M. Magnetic resonance imaging of the elbow. Part II: Abnormalities of the ligaments, tendons, and nerves. Skeletal Radiol 2005; 34(1):1–18.
60. Giuffre BM, Moss MJ. Optimal positioning for MRI of the distal biceps brachii tendon: flexed abducted supinated view. AJR Am J Roentgenol 2004;182(4): 944–6.
61. Liessi G, Cesari S, Spaliviero B, et al. CT and MR findings of cubital bursitis: a report of five cases. Skeletal Radiol 1996;25(5):471–5.
62. Miller TT, Adler RS. Sonography of tears of the distal biceps tendon. AJR Am J Roentgenol 2000;175(4):1081–6.
63. Tagliafico A, Michaud J, Capaccio E, et al. Ultrasound demonstration of distal biceps tendon bifurcation: normal and abnormal findings. Eur Radiol 2010; 20(1):202–8.
64. Giuffre BM, Lisle DA. Tear of the distal biceps branchii tendon: a new method of ultrasound evaluation. Australas Radiol 2005;49(5):404–6.
65. Kalume Brigido M, De Maeseneer M, Jacobson JA, et al. Improved visualization of the radial insertion of the biceps tendon at ultrasound with a lateral approach. Eur Radiol 2009;19(7):1817–21.
66. Levy M, Fishel RE, Stern GM. Triceps tendon avulsion with or without fracture of the radial head–a rare injury? J Trauma 1978;18(9):677–9.

67. Rood LK, Hevesy GZ. An unusual complication of radial head fractures. Am J Emerg Med 1991;9(6):553–4.

68. Mair SD, Isbell WM, Gill TJ, et al. Triceps tendon ruptures in professional football players. Am J Sports Med 2004;32(2):431–4.

69. Duchow J, Kelm J, Kohn D. Acute ulnar nerve compression syndrome in a powerlifter with triceps tendon rupture–a case report. Int J Sports Med 2000;21(4):308–10.

70. Sollender JL, Rayan GM, Barden GA. Triceps tendon rupture in weight lifters. J Shoulder Elbow Surg 1998;7(2):151–3.

71. Sierra RJ, Weiss NG, Shrader MW, et al. Acute triceps ruptures: case report and retrospective chart review. J Shoulder Elbow Surg 2006;15(1):130–4.

72. Stannard JP, Bucknell AL. Rupture of the triceps tendon associated with steroid injections. Am J Sports Med 1993;21(3):482–5.

73. de Waal Malefijt MC, Beeker TW. Avulsion of the triceps tendon in secondary hyperparathyroidism. A case report. Acta Orthop Scand 1987;58(4):434–5.

74. Wagner JR, Cooney WP. Rupture of the triceps muscle at the musculotendinous junction: a case report. J Hand Surg Am 1997;22(2):341–3.

75. O'Driscoll SW. Intramuscular triceps rupture. Can J Surg 1992;35(2):203–7.

76. Bos CF, Nelissen RG, Bloem JL. Incomplete rupture of the tendon of triceps brachii. A case report. Int Orthop 1994;18(5):273–5.

77. Keefe DT, Lintner DM. Nerve injuries in the throwing elbow. Clin Sports Med 2004;23(4):723–42, xi.

78. Bordalo-Rodrigues M, Rosenberg ZS. MR imaging of entrapment neuropathies at the elbow. Magn Reson Imaging Clin N Am 2004;12(2):247–63, vi.

79. Andreisek G, Crook DW, Burg D, et al. Peripheral neuropathies of the median, radial, and ulnar nerves: MR imaging features. Radiographics 2006;26(5): 1267–87.

80. Wiesler ER, Chloros GD, Cartwright MS, et al. Ultrasound in the diagnosis of ulnar neuropathy at the cubital tunnel. J Hand Surg Am 2006;31(7):1088–93.

81. Martinoli C, Bianchi S, Zamorani MP, et al. Ultrasound of the elbow. Eur J Ultrasound 2001;14(1):21–7.

82. Martinoli C, Bianchi S, Giovagnorio F, et al. Ultrasound of the elbow. Skeletal Radiol 2001;30(11):605–14.

83. Kinni V, Craig J, van Holsbeeck M, et al. Entrapment of the posterior interosseous nerve at the arcade of Frohse with sonographic, magnetic resonance imaging, and intraoperative confirmation. J Ultrasound Med 2009;28(6):807–12.

84. Husarik DB, Saupe N, Pfirrmann CW, et al. Elbow nerves: MR findings in 60 asymptomatic subjects–normal anatomy, variants, and pitfalls. Radiology 2009;252(1):148–56.

85. Bladt L, Vankan Y, Demeyere A, et al. Bilateral ulnar nerve compression by anconeus epitrochlearis muscle. JBR-BTR 2009;92(2):120.

86. Dahners LE, Wood FM. Anconeus epitrochlearis, a rare cause of cubital tunnel syndrome: a case report. J Hand Surg Am 1984;9(4):579–80.

87. O'Hara JJ, Stone JH. Ulnar nerve compression at the elbow caused by a prominent medial head of the triceps and an anconeus epitrochlearis muscle. J Hand Surg Br 1996;21(1):133–5.

88. Hayashi Y, Kojima T, Kohno T. A case of cubital tunnel syndrome caused by the snapping of the medial head of the triceps brachii muscle. J Hand Surg Am 1984;9(1):96–9.

89. Gervasio O, Zaccone C. Surgical approach to ulnar nerve compression at the elbow caused by the epitrochleoanconeus muscle and a prominent medial

head of the triceps. Neurosurgery 2008;62(3 Suppl 1):186–92 [discussion: 192–3].

90. Ochiai N, Honmo J, Tsujino A, et al. Electrodiagnosis in entrapment neuropathy by the arcade of Struthers. Clin Orthop Relat Res 2000;378:129–35.
91. Spinner M, Kaplan EB. The relationship of the ulnar nerve to the medial intermuscular septum in the arm and its clinical significance. Hand 1976;8(3): 239–42.
92. Campbell WW, Pridgeon RM, Sahni SK. Entrapment neuropathy of the ulnar nerve at its point of exit from the flexor carpi ulnaris muscle. Muscle Nerve 1988;11(5):467–70.
93. Amadio PC, Beckenbaugh RD. Entrapment of the ulnar nerve by the deep flexor-pronator aponeurosis. J Hand Surg Am 1986;11(1):83–7.
94. Lordan J, Rauh P, Spinner RJ. The clinical anatomy of the supracondylar spur and the ligament of Struthers. Clin Anat 2005;18(7):548–51.
95. Aydinlioglu A, Cirak B, Akpinar F, et al. Bilateral median nerve compression at the level of Struthers' ligament. Case report. J Neurosurg 2000;92(4):693–6.
96. Bilge T, Yalaman O, Bilge S, et al. Entrapment neuropathy of the median nerve at the level of the ligament of Struthers. Neurosurgery 1990;27(5):787–9.
97. Martinelli P, Gabellini AS, Poppi M, et al. Pronator syndrome due to thickened bicipital aponeurosis. J Neurol Neurosurg Psychiatry 1982;45(2):181–2.
98. Tsai P, Steinberg DR. Median and radial nerve compression about the elbow. Instr Course Lect 2008;57:177–85.
99. Javeed N, Javeed H, Javeed S, et al. Anterior interosseous nerve syndrome due to aneurysm of arterio-venous fistula. J Clin Rheumatol 1997;3(3):147.
100. Proudman TW, Menz PJ. An anomaly of the median artery associated with the anterior interosseous nerve syndrome. J Hand Surg Br 1992;17(5):507–9.
101. Nigst H, Dick W. Syndromes of compression of the median nerve in the proximal forearm (pronator teres syndrome; anterior interosseous nerve syndrome). Arch Orthop Trauma Surg 1979;93(4):307–12.
102. Dunn AJ, Salonen DC, Anastakis DJ. MR imaging findings of anterior interosseous nerve lesions. Skeletal Radiol 2007;36(12):1155–62.
103. Mitsunaga MM, Nakano K. High radial nerve palsy following strenuous muscular activity. A case report. Clin Orthop Relat Res 1988;234:39–42.
104. Streib E. Upper arm radial nerve palsy after muscular effort: report of three cases. Neurology 1992;42(8):1632–4.
105. Ferdinand BD, Rosenberg ZS, Schweitzer ME, et al. MR imaging features of radial tunnel syndrome: initial experience. Radiology 2006;240(1):161–8.
106. Kijowski R, De Smet AA. MRI findings of osteochondritis dissecans of the capitellum with surgical correlation. AJR Am J Roentgenol 2005;185(6):1453–9.
107. Harada M, Takahara M, Sasaki J, et al. Using sonography for the early detection of elbow injuries among young baseball players. AJR Am J Roentgenol 2006; 187(6):1436–41.

Sports-Related Injuries of the Biceps and Triceps

Gregory I. Bain, MBBS, FRACS, PhD[a,b,*],
Adam W. Durrant, MB, ChB, FRACS[a,b]

KEYWORDS
- Elbow joint • Biceps • Triceps • Rupture • Reconstruction

The biceps and its antagonist, the triceps, are the main flexors and extensors of the elbow joint. In the athlete they are responsible for accelerating the forearm during throwing or pitching and then decelerating the arm to prevent injury to the elbow joint. Rupture of the biceps or triceps is regarded as a rare injury, but in the authors' opinion the incidence appears to be increasing. Historically, operative repair of the biceps brachii was fraught with difficulty, but in recent times surgical techniques have improved and the results of biceps and triceps repair have improved.[1–10]

BICEPS

Distal biceps tendon ruptures are rare, accounting for only 3% to 12% of all biceps tendon injuries. The reported incidence is 1.2 per 100,000 people, the dominant arm being affected 86% of the time. The average age of patients is 50 years old with an age range of 18 to 72 years of age.[2,5,8,11,12] The most commonly cited risk factors are male gender, smoking, anabolic steroid use, and body building.[11–13] The proposed etiologies are manyfold; the most commonly implicated include an irregularity of the radial tuberosity, radial bursitis, and a watershed area of poor arterial supply.[14–17] Tears within the substance of the tendon or at its musculotendinous junction are rare, with the vast majority of tears occurring at the distal insertion.[18,19]

ANATOMY

Compared with the anatomy and physiology of the proximal end of the biceps muscle, the anatomy of the distal biceps tendon was poorly understood; however, in recent

a Orthopaedic Department, Modbury Hospital, Smart Road, Modbury, South Australia 5092, Australia
b Department of Orthopaedic Surgery, University of Adelaide, Royal Adelaide Hospital, North Terrace, South Australia 5001, Australia
* Corresponding author. 196 Melbourne Street, North Adelaide, SA 5006, Australia.
E-mail address: greg@gregbain.com.au

Clin Sports Med 29 (2010) 555–576
doi:10.1016/j.csm.2010.07.002
0278-5919/10/$ – see front matter © 2010 Elsevier Inc. All rights reserved.

sportsmed.theclinics.com

years our understanding has improved.[20] Most anatomic descriptions have suggested that the muscle originates as 2 proximal heads that merge at the level of the deltoid tuberosity to form a single muscle belly.[21] In work undertaken by Eames and colleagues,[20] this was not found to be the case. In 10 of 17 specimens they dissected, they found that the short head (originating from the coracoid process) and the long head (originating from the superior lip of the glenoid) continued along their entire length as separate muscles. Each muscle was surrounded by loose epimysial tissue and the short head remained on the ulnar side of the arm throughout its course, with the long head running parallel to it. In the remaining 7 specimens there was varying amounts of interdigitation of the muscle into a raphe in the distal third of the muscle bellies. This interdigitation is usually easily separated with the gloved finger.

At the level of the lacertus fibrosus, the tendons continue in line with their respective muscle bellies and may be separate or fuse into one structure. If the tendons do combine, they are still easily dissected into their separate bundles. The lacertus fibrosus itself arises at the level of the musculotendinous junction. It consists of 3 layers, which are postulated to play a role in stabilizing the tendon distally.[20,22]

The long head tendon inserts onto the prominence of the radial tuberosity. The short head attaches more distally onto the shaft of the radius. It is interesting to note the position of the two insertions relative to the axis of forearm rotation, which extends from the center of the capitellum to the center of the head of the ulna. By inserting into the prominence of the radial tuberosity, the long head of biceps positions itself at the maximum distance that the radius extends from the axis of rotation of the forearm, thus providing maximal rotatory torque. The short head inserts predominantly along the line of the center of rotation of the forearm, thereby providing greater flexion leverage and a reduced rotation torque.[20]

Eames and Bain[20] further divide the distal biceps tendon into 3 zones:

Zone 1, *preaponeurosis*: a variable amount of muscular interdigitation of the two bellies occurs, with many cadavers showing none at all.

Zone 2, *aponeurosis or lacertus fibrosus*: the lacertus fibrosus consists of 3 layers and has a wide and deep involvement in the flexor compartment of the forearm; it completely encircles the flexors and has fascial attachments particularly to the ulnar flexors, and incorporates the median nerve and brachial artery.

Zone 3, *postaponeurosis*: the two tendons continue distally past lacertus fibrosus and insert onto the radial tuberosity.

Etiology

Local degenerative and pathologic changes are thought to be a factor in the etiology of acute ruptures of the distal biceps tendon. These changes include hypertrophic changes of the radial tuberosity,[14,17] which lead to abrasion of the tendon during rotatory movements and biceps bursitis.[23] Theories have also included hypovascularity of the tendon adjacent to the insertion of the radial tuberosity.[17] When the forearm rotates, the space between the radius and ulna is narrowed, which could abrade or compress the biceps tendon during the repeated forearm rotation.[8,14] Synovitis or osseous lipping can narrow this gap resulting in compression and direct attrition of the tendon. As with other tendons, anabolic steroid use among body builders has also been implicated in acute biceps tendon rupture, but body building in isolation is also thought to be a risk factor. There is a higher incidence of distal biceps tendon rupture in males, but this statistic may be biased because of the higher rates of men being employed in occupations involving heavy lifting. It is also thought that there is a higher incidence in smokers. The dominant arm is affected 86% of the time.[12]

During power grip there is proximal migration of the forearm musculature that puts increased tension on the lacertus fibrosis, which in turn pulls the biceps tendon in an ulnar direction and increases the force of, and on, the biceps tendon. This point is important physiologically for providing a supramaximal force, but also becomes an etiologic factor in acute tendon ruptures (**Fig. 1**).[18]

Clinical Presentation

A typical history is for male patients to describe a sudden episode of severe pain while performing a forced eccentric contraction of the biceps.[3,16] Occasionally, they will also describe hearing a pop or snap in the region of the elbow. This is followed by an immediate loss of elbow flexion power or even a complete pseudoparalysis.[3,5,11,12] Patients will typically have ecchymosis on the medial aspect of the elbow that may extend proximally and distally (**Fig. 2**). This finding is not consistent, as an intact lacertus fibrosus may confine the hematoma and thus prevent ecchymosis formation, particularly in a partial rupture.[4] In a complete rupture there will be a palpable defect or emptiness of the antecubital fossa, which is not present when there is a partial rupture.[2,16,18] There will be pain and weakness with flexion and supination of the elbow against resistance. With proximal migration of the biceps muscular-tendinous unit, there may be an abnormal contour of the biceps muscle with an increased prominence on the anteromedial aspect, the so-called Popeye deformity.[2,4,8,9,12,15,24] In partial tears there will not be proximal migration of the muscular-tendinous unit, therefore no deformity will be present. If a large bursitis is present, then compression of the median nerve can occur.[25]

The hook test, as described by O'Driscoll and colleagues,[26] can be used to assess for continuity of the biceps tendon. The examiners finger is placed on the lateral boarder of the antecubital fossa and then a force is applied into the fossa directed medially, trying to hook under the biceps tendon. If the tendon is intact, the examiners finger meets resistance and the tip can be introduced partially under the tendon, demonstrating its patency (**Fig. 3**).

The authors preferred technique is to passively supinate and pronate the forearm with the elbow at 90° of flexion. In the intact biceps tendon, this passive motion will be accompanied by visible pistonlike movements of the biceps muscle belly, which will be absent if there is a complete rupture of the biceps tendon. In patients with a partial tear, the muscle will still piston; however, there will be pain or weakness of supination against resistance. In patients with a traumatic episode and anterior elbow pain, this is important to assess.

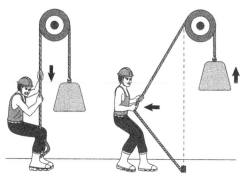

Fig. 1. Ulnar pull of the biceps tendon by the lacertus fibrosus increases the pull of the distal biceps tendon.

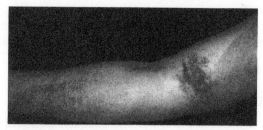

Fig. 2. Ecchymosis following biceps tendon rupture. (*Reproduced from* Bain GI. Repair of distal biceps tendon avulsion with the Endobutton technique. Techniques in Shoulder & Elbow Surgery 2002;3(2):96–101; with permission.)

INVESTIGATIONS
Radiograph

Plain radiographs usually do not identify any other abnormality other than maybe some soft-tissue swelling. A rupture with a degenerative etiology may reveal some calcific changes at the radial tuberosity, but this is certainly not a reliable diagnostic finding. Calcific changes have only been reported in complete ruptures of the distal biceps tendon, but have yet to be reported in partial tears.

MRI

The MRI scanner can be used to demonstrate the biceps tendon. Traditionally, scanning of the distal biceps tendon has been undertaken in the axial plane, with the patients' arm extended.[27,28] Because of the oblique course of the tendon in the antecubital fossa to its insertion on the radial tuberosity, longitudinal views are often difficult to obtain, which makes diagnosis of partial tears particularly difficult to diagnose as it may be confused with tendinitis.

Giuffre and Moss[28] described a method for optimal patient positioning that allows for full length views of the biceps brachii tendon from the musculotendinous junction to its insertion on the radial tuberosity in at least 1, if not 2, sections. Patients are positioned prone in the scanner with the affected arm above their head (shoulder abducted 180° with the arm beside the head and elbow flexed 90° with the forearm supinated and the thumb pointing upwards). This position has become known as the *FABS* (Flexion, Abduction, Supination) position and is enhanced by placing a shoulder phased array coil around the elbow so that it becomes the center-of-magnet position. The FABS sequence is combined with conventional views of the biceps brachii (**Figs. 4** and **5**).

Ultrasound

Ultrasonography has been used extensively to aid in the diagnosis of biceps tendon rupture because it is cheaper than MRI, is available at most hospitals, and can be performed in most clinical circumstances. It can be used to confirm the continuity of the distal tendon or perceived changes in caliber of the tendinous structure.[27] Dynamic ultrasound can also be used to help differentiate partial from complete tears of the distal biceps tendon. Peritendinous fluid, such as blood or edema, can also be visualized. Ultrasonography is made difficult when the tissues are thick, such as in obese or muscular patients or those with previous surgery to the tendon. Unfortunately it is highly operator dependant and less reproducible than MRI. Ultrasound assessment requires an experienced musculoskeletal ultrasonographer. Bird[29] developed the

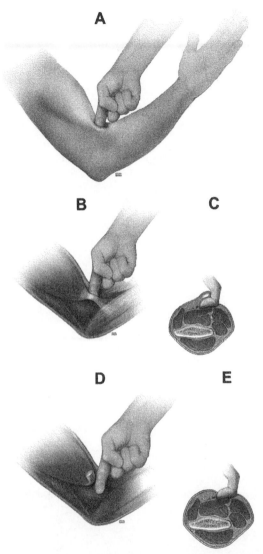

Fig. 3. (*A*) Hook test as described by SW O'Driscoll and colleagues with elbow flexed to 90° and forearm actively supinated. (*B, C*) Intact tendon. (*D, E*) Complete tear of tendon. (*From* O'Driscoll SW, Goncalves LB, Dietz P. The hook test for distal biceps avulsion. Am J Sports Med 35 2007;(11):1865–9; copyright of Mayo Foundation for Medical Education and Research; with permission.)

use of the pronator teres acoustic window, which can provide a better understanding of the biceps insertion (**Fig. 6**).

Distal Biceps Tendon Endoscopy

Eames and Bain[22] have used biceps bursoscopy to assess patients who have partial tears or biceps bursitis. An incision is made over the distal biceps tendon, and via a mini open approach the arthroscope is introduced into the biceps tendon bursa

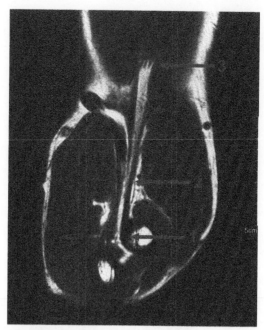

Fig. 4. MRI of normal biceps tendon obtained using FABS view. Arrow 1 points to a radial tuberosity, arrow 2 points to a distal biceps tendon, and arrow 3 points to a musculotendinous junction. Note the brachialis tendon adjacent to the biceps tendon. (*Courtesy of* GI Bain, Adelaide, Australia.)

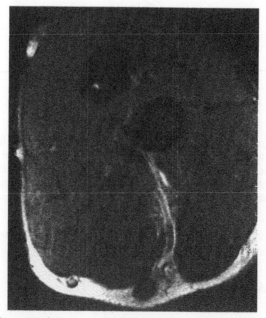

Fig. 5. MRI showing complete tear of biceps tendon. (*Courtesy of* GI Bain, Adelaide, Australia.)

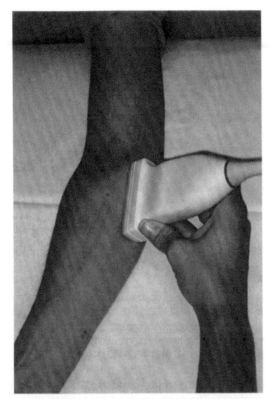

Fig. 6. Ultrasound probe using the pronator window. (*Courtesy of* Steven Bird, Radiographer, Adelaide, Australia.)

(Fig. 7). With this technique the biceps tendon and bursal wall can be assessed as can the proximal shaft of the radius (**Fig. 8**). Partial tears of the biceps tendon and synovitis can be managed with an endoscopic debridement. In view of the close anatomic position of the major neurovascular structures, it is strongly recommended that this first be

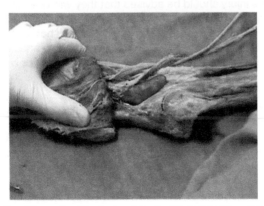

Fig. 7. Cadaveric dissection of a biceps tendon showing the latex injected radiobicipital bursa.

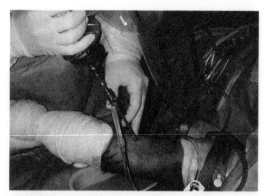

Fig. 8. Biceps bursoscopy with scope introduced with a mini open approach directly into the biceps bursa. (*Reproduced from* Eames MHA, Bain GI. Distal biceps tendon endoscopy and anterior elbow arthroscopy portal. Technique Shoulder Elbow Surg 2006;7(3):139–42; with permission.)

performed in a cadaveric specimen, that the shaver is only turned on when the shaver aperture is clearly in view with the suction off. Conventional nonoperative modalities should have been used before surgical intervention. Patients who are noted at bursoscopy to have significant tears of the tendon (>50%) are managed by completion of the tear and surgical repair. Eames and Bain[22] have also performed an endoscopic debridement of the deep surface of a partial tear of the biceps tendon and then, with an endoscopic-assisted procedure, performed a biceps tendon repair to the bicipital tuberosity footprint. The outer fibers of the tendon were left intact because they were well attached to the periphery of the tuberosity.

MANAGEMENT
Nonoperative

Tears of the distal biceps tendon can be managed nonoperatively. The ideal patients for this are those who have an essentially sedentary job, or who have medical comorbidities that preclude an anesthetic. Patients who elect to have nonoperative management of their biceps injury should be advised that they will lose between 20% to 55% of supination strength and 62% of supination endurance, and 8% to 36% of flexion strength and 86% of flexion endurance.[4,5,8,16,18,30] They should also be advised that there will be a contour difference between the biceps of the affected and unaffected sides. Physiotherapy may help to strengthen the secondary elbow flexors.

Surgical Repair of Complete Tears

In view of the fact that the natural history provided by nonoperative management is to continue to have marked weakness, particularly with supination, surgical repair is recommended in the majority of patients.[2,3,5,8,16.] Historically, the 2-incision technique was developed because of the concern regarding the anterior exposure and risk of injury of the radial nerve.[31] With the 2-incision technique there has been several reports of radioulnar synostosis, which has not been reported using a single anterior incision.[2,8,15,16] In those patients where a radioulnar synostosis does occur, excision is usually required. Unfortunately, the distal biceps tendon is usually incorporated in the synostosis and may require repair after removal of the synostosis.[18,31]

There are several different fixation methods that can be used. The use of suture anchors has been used by some authors because of their simplicity of insertion.[32] However, biomechanical studies demonstrate that there is a superior pull out strength using an EndoButton technique (440 N) than suture anchors (381 N), bone tunnel (310 N), and interference fit screws (232 N).[6,7,33] The EndoButton (Acufex, Acufex Microsurgical, Mansfield, MA, USA) is robust and has holes large enough to accommodate the number 5 Ethibond (Ethicon, San Angelo, TX, USA) suture. The stronger fixation allows early active mobilization.[2]

Technique

Patients are given a general anesthetic and a 5-cm longitudinal incision is made from the elbow skin crease distally. Care is taken to ensure that the lateral cutaneous nerve of the forearm is protected. With the elbow held in full extension and supination, the radial tuberosity can be palpated in the forearm. In an acute case, full formal exposure of the major neurovascular structures is not required.

Handheld retractors are used to expose the radial tuberosity. The authors recommend not using lever retractors, such as Hohmann retractors, because these may lead to neurovascular complications caused by their increased force.[2] In the upper arm, the biceps tendon is palpated and delivered into the wound. A cortical window large enough to accommodate the biceps tendon is made on the proximal radius with the aid of a high-speed burr. It is important to have the arm in full supination and to place this cortical window as medially as possible to try and recreate the position of the anatomic insertion of the biceps tendon onto the bicipital tuberosity.

A 4.5-mm drill is advanced through to the posterior cortex of the proximal radius. A drill guide is used to protect the anterior soft-tissue structures. A cadaveric study has demonstrated a safe zone of 30° from the vertical plane when drilling into the radius with the forearm in supination to prevent injury to the posterior interosseous nerve. (**Figs. 9** and **10**).[2]

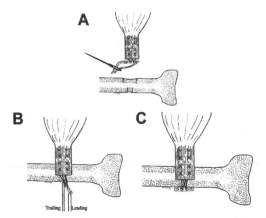

Fig. 9. (*A*) Straight-eyed needle with leading and trailing sutures. (*B*) Endobutton advances tendon into intramedullary canal of radius under fluoroscopic control. (*C*) Endobutton locks tendon into position, and trailing sutures are removed. (*Reprinted from* Bain GI, Prem H, Heptinstall RJ, et al. Repair of distal biceps tendon rupture: a new technique using the Endobutton. J Shoulder Elbow Surg 2000;9(2):120–6; with permission.)

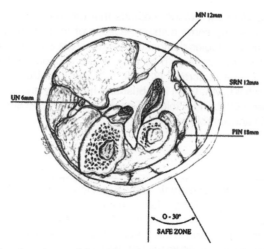

Fig. 10. Cross-sectional anatomy of forearm at level of radial tuberosity with relationship of major nerves. MN, median nerve (just proximal teres muscle); PIN, posterior interosseous nerve (anteriorly at the arcade of Frohse); SBRN, superficial branch of radial nerve; UN, ulnar nerve. (*Reprinted from* Bain GI, Prem H, Heptinstall RJ, et al. Repair of distal biceps tendon rupture: a new technique using the Endobutton. J Shoulder Elbow Surg 2000;9(2):120–6; with permission.)

A Number 5 Ethibond Bunnell suture is placed into the biceps tendon. The sutures are advanced down to the end of the tendon and advanced through the middle 2 holes of the Endobutton (**Fig. 11**). The sutures are tied proximally so that they do not impinge when locking the EndoButton. Sutures are also placed into the leading and trailing holes of the EndoButton. These sutures are placed through the eye of a straight needle or Beath Pin, which is then advanced through the hole in the shaft of the radius and

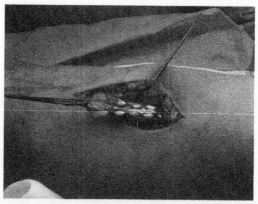

Fig. 11. Biceps tendon is delivered through an anterior incision and the Endobutton is attached with 2 Bunnell, number 5 Ethibond sutures. Leading and trailing sutures are attached to the outer holes of the Endobutton, thereby preparing it for insertion. (*Courtesy of* A. Durrant and GI Bain, Adelaide, Australia.)

withdrawn from the posterior aspect. This procedure delivers the sutures through the drill holes in the radius. The elbow is placed into a flexed and supinated position and the EndoButton is advanced by placing traction on the sutures. The leading and trailing sutures can then be manipulated, like the strings of a puppet, to advance the EndoButton through the radius. The final position of the EndoButton on the dorsal cortex of the radius should be confirmed with fluoroscopy.

Rehabilitation

Rehabilitation of patients depends on the repair technique used. Because of the high pull-out strength of the EndoButton technique, patients are advised that they can remove the arm from the sling in the first week but not to do any heavy lifting or grasping for a period of 3 months.

Partial Distal Biceps Tendon Rupture

Assessment and management of these patients can be difficult. Patients will often give a history of an eccentric injury to the elbow. Patients will have localized tenderness over the anterior aspect of the elbow, weakness of supination, and flexion against resistance. Imaging in the form of ultrasound and MRI scan can be difficult to interpret. However, echogenic changes in the biceps tendon and associated effusion of the bicipital bursa is often identified.

Although it is generally agreed that complete tears of the distal biceps tendon require immediate surgical repair to maximize functional outcomes, the same may not be true of partial tears.[3–7,18] The literature currently states that tears less than 50% of the total insertional footprint do not require surgical reattachment.[22,25] Tears involving greater than 50% of the insertional footprint require formal surgical division and reattachment using standard techniques.[18,22,25,26,34–36] What is not yet known is the functional outcomes of tears of long head versus short head with regards to operative versus nonoperative management.[18] Eames and Bain[22] used biceps endoscopy to further classify biceps tendon injuries and to help guide treatment (**Fig. 12, Table 1**).

The authors have had 3 patients in which one head of the biceps tendon was avulsed, which has been the tendon of the larger short head. The long head was intact. Endoscopy is useful to confirm this. The authors have reattached the torn head using the EndoButton technique.

Delayed Presentation Distal Biceps Tendon Rupture

Delayed presentation of a distal biceps tendon rupture poses a difficult operative reconstruction problem to the surgeon. Usually the tendon has retracted proximomedial into the brachium and it is not possible to pull it out to length for direct repair. Various techniques have been described to try and gain length from the tendon, such as slides of the biceps brachii and fractional lengthening of the remaining tendon. Most of these techniques are difficult to perform and do not provide a satisfactory repair.

The remaining biceps tendon can also be directly sutured to the tendon of the brachialis muscle. This is a nonanatomic repair (or tenodesis) and does little to address the loss of supination strength.

Reconstruction of the biceps tendon is the preferred option. An option is to use autograft hamstring tendon grafts to reconstruct the delayed presentation biceps tendon rupture. The patients' semitendinosus tendon is harvested using the same technique as used for an anterior cruciate ligament reconstruction. The autograft tendon is folded at its midpoint and both free ends are then woven through the biceps tendon stump using tendon passers. The weave is reinforced by suturing the autograft in place. Number 5 Ethibond or a similar heavy grade suture are passed in a Bunnell

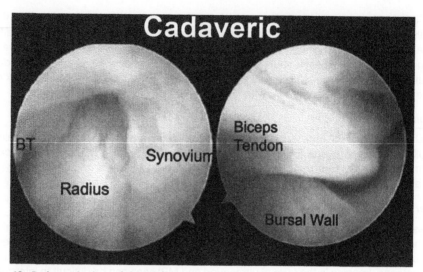

Fig. 12. Endoscopic view of the biceps tendon and bursa. (*From* Eames MHA, Bain GI. Distal biceps tendon endoscopy and anterior elbow arthroscopy portal. Tech Shoulder Elbow Surg 2006;7(3):139–42; with permission.)

fashion through the autograft-biceps tendon construct and secured to an EndoButton (**Figs. 13** and **14**). The free end of the autograft is then secured to the proximal radius in the same fashion as that used for a primary repair.[37] Another option is to use the allograft hamstring tendon.

Morrey[15,16] described the use of an Achilles tendon allograft. The tendinous portion of the graft is teased out into a flat sheet, which is wrapped around the biceps tendon as a sleeve and then sutured in place. The bone block from the calcaneus is then seated into the proximal radius and sutured into place. This technique provides a reliable way of regaining length in the biceps tendon and if the allograft bone graft incorporates, a strong bond to the proximal radius. It is the authors' experience that the allograft Achilles tendon is easy to wrap around the biceps muscle, but it is difficult to secure to the muscle. If patients request an allograft, the authors prefer to use allograft hamstring tendon, which is weaved through the tendon stump and the distal biceps muscle. This procedure provides a strong, secure fixation of the tendon.

TRICEPS

Triceps tendon injuries are extremely rare with few reported cases in the literature. There is a male predominance (2:1, male to female) and a wide age range in which the injuries occur.[38] The first published case report of a triceps tendon rupture was by Partridge in 1868.[10] Anzel reviewed the Mayo Clinic experience with more than 1000 tendon injuries. He found that approximately 0.8% were triceps injuries, and half of those were caused by open lacerations to the posterior aspect of the upper arm.[1] In the North American National Football League there were only 21 cases of triceps tendon rupture over a 6-year period.[39] This figure is possibly not a true representation of the incidence in the general population because there is an increased incidence of tendon ruptures in contact sports, probably because of the violent nature of

Table 1
Classification of insertional (zone 3) distal biceps tendon injury

Grade	Injury	Signs		Treatment
Grade 0	Distal biceps tendinosis	Pain on resisted supination and flexion		Nonoperative
Grade 1	Distal biceps tendon partial tear	Pain and weakness on resisted supination and flexion		Biceps endoscopy
Grade 2	Combined short and long head avulsion, lacertus intact, minimal muscle retraction	Marked weakness of resisted supination and flexion Positive hook test		Biceps tendon repair
Grade 3	Complete tendon rupture with torn lacertus fibrosus and muscle retraction	Marked weakness of resisted supination and flexion Positive hook test Empty cubital fossa		Biceps tendon repair ± lacertus repair
Grade 4	Delayed presentation	Persistent weakness of resisted supination and flexion Positive hook test Proximal retraction of muscle belly		Autograft or allograft reconstruction procedure

Adapted from Bain GI, Johnson L, Watts AC. Endoscopic distal biceps repair. In: Savoie FH, Field LD, editors. AANA advanced arthroscopy: the elbow and wrist. Philadelphia: Saunders-Elsevier; 2010; with permission.

the sports, but also because of the potential for steroid use among professional athletes.[38,39] In adolescents, avulsions of the olecranon apophysis can occur, detaching the triceps insertion to the olecranon; however, this is not a true tendon rupture. The apophysis may still need reattachment.[40]

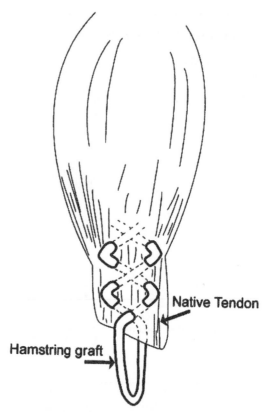

Fig. 13. The Hamstring autograft is interwoven into the biceps tendon. (*Reprinted from* Hallam P, Bain GI. Repair of chronic distal biceps tendon ruptures using autologous hamstring graft and the Endobutton. J Shoulder Elbow Surg 2004;13(6):648–51; with permission.)

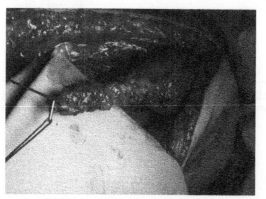

Fig. 14. Hamstring autograft-bicep tendon complex with Endobutton attached. (*Reprinted from* Hallam P, Bain GI. Repair of chronic distal biceps tendon ruptures using autologous hamstring graft and the Endobutton. J Shoulder Elbow Surg 2004;13(6):648–51; with permission.)

ANATOMY

The triceps brachii is made up of 3 muscle bellies. The infraglenoid tubercle of the scapula gives rise to the long head. The medial head arises from the posterior aspect of the distal humerus distal to the spiral groove and is muscular almost until the triceps insertion. The lateral head arises from the lateral intermuscular septum and the posterolateral aspect of the humerus above the spiral groove.[21] In some cadaveric specimens there is a fourth head, the dorsal epitrochlearis, which arises from the posteromedial humerus between the triceps proper and the latissimus dorsi.

The triceps inserts as a bilaminate tendon into an area on the tip of the olecranon over a wide area that also blends with the posterior capsule of the elbow joint. The width of the distal triceps tendon varies from 19 mm to 42 mm, the insertion footprint averaging 466 mm^2.[38] The medial aspect of the triceps insertion is along the crest of the ulna. The lateral triceps expansion is analogous to the lacertus fibrosus of the biceps brachii in that it has a wide insertion to the fascia of the extensor carpi ulnaris muscle, the anconeus, and also into the antebrachial fascia of the forearm.[38]

Mechanism of Injury

Triceps injuries most commonly occur as the result of a fall on the outstretched hand, resulting in an extended elbow that is suddenly decelerated. The tear is most commonly at the insertion of the tendon.[41] Tears at the musculotendinous junction are extremely rare[42] as are those that occur within the muscle belly.[43,44] It is not uncommon for patients to suffer associated injuries, such as a fractured radial head or wrist. Numerous associations have been observed; however, because of the low prevalence of the condition these factors cannot be defined as causative. Conditions that have been implicated include body building,[45] anabolic steroid use,[46] hyperparathyroidism,[47] local steroid injection,[46] renal osteodystrophy,[48] olecranon bursitis,[49] osteogenesis inperfecta,[50] and systemic lupus erythematosus.[51] Injuries to the triceps tendon can also be associated with direct penetrating trauma to the triceps muscle or tendon.[52] As with biceps tendon ruptures, there is also an association with body building and power lifting, but again this may be caused by anabolic steroid abuse.[45,53]

Presentation

Patients will indicate pain in the region of the olecranon at the site of the triceps insertion with pain on palpation at the indicated site. There will usually be a palpable defect in the tendon. Some patients may not have noticed a weakness of elbow extension as anconeus, aided by gravity, can substitute for the triceps, especially when the activities are below shoulder height. With this in mind, triceps power should be assessed with the affected arm held overhead and patients asked to extend the elbow, first against gravity and then against resistance. Even with anconeus activity, the triceps will test weak against resistance.

Examination may reveal ecchymosis over the posterior aspect of the upper arm and a palpable gap just proximal to the olecranon process. This gap may not be easily appreciated if there is considerable swelling or if patients are obese.[38] A modification of the Thompson squeeze test used to diagnose Achilles tendon ruptures has been reported. Patients are positioned prone with the elbow flexed and the forearm over the side of the table. The triceps bulk is then squeezed, an intact tendon will result in some extension of the elbow.[54,55]

Investigations

Plain film radiographs are not particularly useful, but may aid in the diagnosis of a ruptured triceps mechanism if an avulsed fleck of bone is noted posterior to the distal humerus, which is known as the *fleck sign* (**Fig. 15**).[42,56] The other area where plain films are useful is to aid in the diagnosis of injuries associated with triceps rupture, such as ipsilateral radial head and distal radius fractures. MRI is the best technique for assessment of the injury because it provides the clinician with more information as to the site of the injury (insertional, musculotendinous, or intramuscular) and if it is a partial or complete rupture of the tendon.[38,56,57] In centers where MRI is not readily available, ultrasound can be used as an alternative to help confirm triceps tendon rupture.

Treatment

The treatment of acute tears of the triceps needs to be guided by the site of the rupture, the delay to treatment, and the functional demands or expectations of the patients.[58] Acute tears (<2 weeks old) can usually be repaired directly, and even those considerably older may be amenable to a direct repair. Chronic ruptures may require reconstruction. Partial tears, like those of the biceps tendon, remain an area of contention as to how they should be managed.

Several techniques are reported in the literature for the repair of the acute triceps tendon rupture. These techniques include the use of transosseous tunnels, suture anchors, interference screws, or a combination of these techniques (**Fig. 16**).[8,38,39,45,50,53,56,58–60] If a large fragment of bone has been avulsed, this may be amenable to direct repair using a cancellous screw over a washer. It is the authors' opinion that this should be reinforced with transosseous sutures. A recent technique described by Yeh and colleagues[38] uses a combination of a grasping stitch in the tendon and then suture anchors in a suture-bridge fashion to recreate the triceps tendon footprint on the olecranon.

Chronic ruptures (>6 weeks from injury) represent a more challenging clinical problem. Often direct repair is not possible and a reconstructive procedure must be

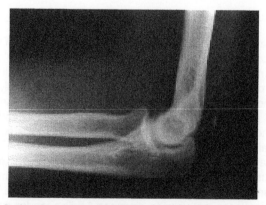

Fig. 15. Radiograph showing avulsed fragment of bone from olecranon. Image: triceps rupture. (*From* Rajasekhar C, Kakarlapudi TK, Bhamra MS. Avulsion of the triceps tendon. Emerg Med J 2002;19:271–2; copyright 2002 from BMJ Publishing Group Ltd; with permission.)

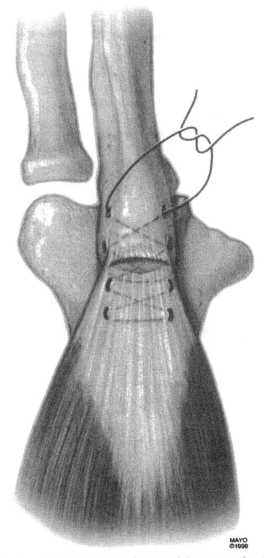

Fig. 16. Repair of ruptured triceps tendon to bone with heavy nonabsorbable suture (eg, 5 Ethibond) through drill holes. Image: repair to bone. (*From* Morrey BF. Radial head fractures. In: Morrey BF, editor. The elbow and its disorders. 3rd edition. Philadelphia: W.B. Saunders Company; copyright 2000, Mayo Foundation for Medical Education and Research, all rights reserved; with permission.)

employed. If the defect is large, the surgeon may need to consider the use of a ligament augmentation to bridge the gap between the end of the torn tendon and olecranon.[58,61,62] The authors' preference is to use an autogenous hamstring graft woven into the triceps stump and then secured through drill holes either with an interference fit screw or sutures (**Fig. 17**). The use of an Achilles osteotendinous allograft has also been described.[58]

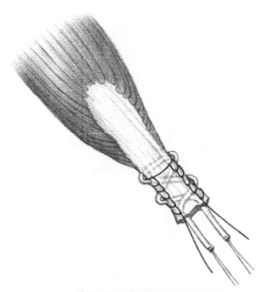

Fig. 17. Ligament augmentation device interwoven through triceps tendon. Image: ligament augmentation device. (*From* Morrey BF. Radial head fractures. In: Morrey BF, editor. The elbow and its disorders. 3rd edition. Philadelphia: W.B. Saunders Company; copyright 2000, Mayo Foundation for Medical Education and Research, all rights reserved; with permission.)

If the tendon has not retracted too far, an anconeus slide can be performed. The anconeus is mobilized from its insertion and attached to the olecranon and the distal end of the torn triceps tendon is attached to the medial border of the anconeus (**Fig. 18**).[63]

It is difficult to find any objective data in the literature regarding the outcomes of triceps repairs. Most investigators describe their results as very good to excellent, and most papers offer a retrospective review using range of motion as their surrogate measures of function.[39,42,53,55,64] Even more lacking is the results of any reconstructions, probably because of the small numbers treated by any one author, and the differing techniques in use. Van Riet is the only investigator to review his results of reconstructions, he found that in 9 subjects, the average strength of the reconstructed side was 66% compared with the contralateral triceps.[41]

THE SNAPPING TRICEPS TENDON

A snapping elbow is a sensation caused by a portion of the triceps mechanism and may be confused with subluxation of the ulnar nerve over the medial epicondyle of the humerus on flexion and extension of the elbow.[65,66] It is caused either by an abnormal medial triceps insertion, an aberrant triceps tendon, or cubitus varus and is typically present with concurrent irritation of the ulnar nerve.[67] Surgical management is only required if patients do not tolerate the symptoms and are directed at the cause. The dislocating portion of the triceps may be mobilized and transferred under the distal triceps and attached to the lateral attachment of the triceps; the aberrant tendon

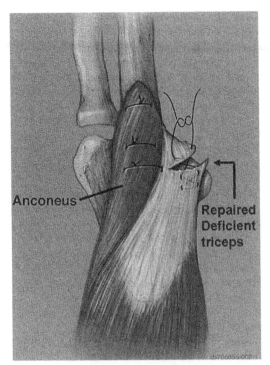

Fig. 18. Anconeus slide. The anconeus is detached and then attached to the olecranon by tenodesis. The triceps is reinforced to the medial border of anconeus. Image: anconeus slide. (*From* Morrey BF. Radial head fractures. In: Morrey BF, editor. The elbow and its disorders. 3rd edition. Philadelphia: W.B. Saunders Company; copyright 2000, Mayo Foundation for Medical Education and Research, all rights reserved; with permission.)

can be excised or distal humerus osteotomy performed to correct deformity. Decompression and transposition of the ulnar nerve may also be indicated.

REFERENCES

1. Anzel SH, Covey KW, Weiner AD, et al. Disruption of muscles and tendons; an analysis of 1,014 cases. Surgery 1959;45(3):406–14.
2. Bain GI, Prem H, Heptinstall RJ, et al. Repair of distal biceps tendon rupture: a new technique using the Endobutton. J Shoulder Elbow Surg 2000;9(2):120–6.
3. Baker BE, Bierwagen D. Rupture of the distal tendon of the biceps brachii. Operative versus non-operative treatment. J Bone Joint Surg Am 1985;67(3):414–7.
4. Bernstein AD, Breslow MJ, Jazrawi LM. Distal biceps tendon ruptures: a historical perspective and current concepts. Am J Orthop (Belle Mead NJ) 2001;30(3): 193–200.
5. Chavan PR, Duquin TR, Bisson LJ. Repair of the ruptured distal biceps tendon: a systematic review. Am J Sports Med 2008;36(8):1618–24.
6. Greenberg JA, Fernandez JJ, Wang T, et al. EndoButton-assisted repair of distal biceps tendon ruptures. J Shoulder Elbow Surg 2003;12(5):484–90.
7. Greenberg JA, Fernandez JJ, Wang T, et al. Erratum from EndoButton assisted repair of distal biceps tendon ruptures. J Shoulder Elbow Surg 2005;14(2):231.

8. Johnson DC, Allen AA. Biceps and triceps tendon injury. In: Altchek DW, Andrews JR, editors. The athlete's elbow. Hagerstown (MD): Lippincott Williams & Wilkins; 2001. p. 105–20.
9. McReynolds IS. Avulsion of the insertion of the biceps brachii tendon and its surgical treatment. J Bone Joint Surg 1963;45A:1780–1.
10. Partridge. A case of rupture of the triceps cubiti. Med Times Gaz 1868;1:175.
11. D'Alessandro DF, Shields CL Jr, Tibone JE, et al. Repair of distal biceps tendon ruptures in athletes. Am J Sports Med 1993;21(1):114–9.
12. Safran MR, Graham SM. Distal biceps tendon ruptures: incidence, demographics, and the effect of smoking. Clin Orthop Relat Res 2002;404:275–83.
13. Visuri T, Lindholm H. Bilateral distal biceps tendon avulsions with use of anabolic steroids. Med Sci Sports Exerc 1994;26(8):941–4.
14. Davis WM, Yassine Z. An etiological factor in tear of the distal tendon of the biceps brachii; report of two cases. J Bone Joint Surg Am 1956;38-A(6):1365–8.
15. Morrey BF. Biceps tendon injury. Instr Course Lect 1999;48:405–10.
16. Morrey BF. Distal biceps tendon rupture. In: Morrey BF, editor. The elbow. Hagerstown (MD): Lippincott Williams & Wilkins; 2001. p. 173–91.
17. Seiler JG 3rd, Parker LM, Chamberland PD, et al. The distal biceps tendon. Two potential mechanisms involved in its rupture: arterial supply and mechanical impingement. J Shoulder Elbow Surg 1995;4(3):149–56.
18. Bain GI, Johnson LJ, Turner PC. Treatment of partial distal biceps tendon tears. Sports Med Arthrosc 2008;16(3):154–61.
19. Schamblin ML, Safran MR. Injury of the distal biceps at the musculotendinous junction. J Shoulder Elbow Surg 2007;16(2):208–12.
20. Eames MH, Bain GI, Fogg QA, et al. Distal biceps tendon anatomy: a cadaveric study. J Bone Joint Surg Am 2007;89(5):1044–9.
21. Last. Last's anatomy regional and applied. 9th edition. New York: Churchill Livingstone; 1994.
22. Eames MH, Bain GI. Distal biceps tendon endoscopy and anterior elbow arthroscopy portal. Techniques Shoulder Elbow Surg 2006;7(3):139–42.
23. Karanjia ND. Cubital bursitis. J Bone Joint Surg Br 1988;70(5):832–3.
24. Ramsey ML. Distal biceps tendon injuries: diagnosis and management. J Am Acad Orthop Surg 1999;7(3):199–207.
25. Durr HR, Stabler A, Pfahler M, et al. Partial rupture of the distal biceps tendon. Clin Orthop Relat Res 2000;374:195–200.
26. O'Driscoll SW, Goncalves LB, Dietz P. The hook test for distal biceps tendon avulsion. Am J Sports Med 2007;35(11):1865–9.
27. Chew ML, Giuffre BM. Disorders of the distal biceps brachii tendon. Radiographics 2005;25(5):1227–37.
28. Giuffre BM, Moss MJ. Optimal positioning for MRI of the distal biceps brachii tendon: flexed abducted supinated view. AJR Am J Roentgenol 2004;182(4):944–6.
29. Bird S. A new method for ultrasound evaluation of the distal biceps Brachii tendon. Ultrasound Med Biol 2006;32(5S):294 [Official Proceedings of the 11th Congress of the World Federation for Ultrasound in Medicine and Biology, May 2006].
30. Morrey BF, Regan WD. Tendinopathies about the elbow. In: Delee JC, Drez D, editors. Orthopaedic sports medicine: principles and practice, vol. 1. Philadelphia: WB Saunders; 1994. p. 1231–2.
31. Boyd HB, Anderson MD. A method of reinsertion of the distal biceps brachii tendon. J Bone Joint Surg 1961;43A:1041.

32. Barnes SJ, Coleman SG, Gilpin D. Repair of avulsed insertion of biceps. A new technique in four cases. J Bone Joint Surg Br 1993;75(6):938–9.

33. Mazzocca AD, Burton KJ, Romeo AA, et al. Biomechanical evaluation of 4 techniques of distal biceps brachii tendon repair. Am J Sports Med 2007;35(2):252–8.

34. Bourne MH, Morrey BF. Partial rupture of the distal biceps tendon. Clin Orthop Relat Res 1991;271:143–8.

35. Rokito AS, McLaughlin JA, Gallagher MA, et al. Partial rupture of the distal biceps tendon. J Shoulder Elbow Surg 1996;5(1):73–5.

36. Vardakas DG, Musgrave DS, Varitimidis SE, et al. Partial rupture of the distal biceps tendon. J Shoulder Elbow Surg 2001;10(4):377–9.

37. Hallam P, Bain GI. Repair of chronic distal biceps tendon ruptures using autologous hamstring graft and the Endobutton. J Shoulder Elbow Surg 2004;13(6):648–51.

38. Yeh PC, Dodds SD, Smart LR, et al. Distal triceps rupture. J Am Acad Orthop Surg 2010;18(1):31–40.

39. Mair SD, Isbell WM, Gill TJ, et al. Triceps tendon ruptures in professional football players. Am J Sports Med 2004;32(2):431–4.

40. Vidal AF, Drakos MC, Allen AA. Biceps tendon and triceps tendon injuries. Clin Sports Med 2004;23(4):707–22, xi.

41. van Riet RP, Morrey BF, Ho E, et al. Surgical treatment of distal triceps ruptures. J Bone Joint Surg Am 2003;85(10):1961–7.

42. Bach BR Jr, Warren RF, Wickiewicz TL. Triceps rupture. A case report and literature review. Am J Sports Med 1987;15(3):285–9.

43. Aso K, Torisu T. Muscle belly tear of the triceps. Am J Sports Med 1984;12(6):485–7.

44. O'Driscoll SW. Intramuscular triceps rupture. Can J Surg 1992;35(2):203–7.

45. Sherman OH, Snyder SJ, Fox JM. Triceps tendon avulsion in a professional body builder. A case report. Am J Sports Med 1984;12(4):328–9.

46. Lambert MI, St Clair GA, Noakes TD. Rupture of the triceps tendon associated with steroid injections. Am J Sports Med 1995;23(6):778.

47. Preston FS, Adicoff A. Hyperparathyroidism with avulsion of three major tendons. Report of a case. N Engl J Med 1962;266:968–71.

48. Mankin HJ. Rickets, osteomalacia, and renal osteodystrophy. Part II. J Bone Joint Surg Am 1974;56(2):352–86.

49. Clayton ML, Thirupathi RG. Rupture of the triceps tendon with olecranon bursitis. A case report with a new method of repair. Clin Orthop Relat Res 1984;184:183–5.

50. Match R, Corrylos E. Bilateral avulsion fracture of the triceps tendon insertion from skiing with osteogenesis imperfecta tarda. Am J Sports Med 1983;11:99–102.

51. Martin JR, Wilson CL, Mathews WH. Bilateral rupture of the ligamenta patellae in a case of disseminated lupus erythematosus. Arthritis Rheum 1958;1(6):548–52.

52. Tarsney FF. Rupture and avulsion of the triceps. Clin Orthop Relat Res 1972;83:177–83.

53. Sollender JL, Rayan GM, Barden GA. Triceps tendon rupture in weight lifters. J Shoulder Elbow Surg 1998;7(2):151–3.

54. Bos CF, Nelissen RG, Bloem JL. Incomplete rupture of the tendon of triceps brachii. A case report. Int Orthop 1994;18(5):273–5.

55. Viegas SF. Avulsion of the triceps tendon. Orthop Rev 1990;19(6):533–6.

56. Pina A, Garcia I, Sabater M. Traumatic avulsion of the triceps brachii. J Orthop Trauma 2002;16:273–6.
57. Kijowski R, Tuite M, Sanford M. Magnetic resonance imaging of the elbow. Part II: Abnormalities of the ligaments, tendons, and nerves. Skeletal Radiol 2005;34(1): 1–18.
58. Morrey BF. Triceps tendon repair and reconstruction. In: Morrey BF, editor. The elbow. Hagerstown (MD): Lippincott Williams & Wilkins; 2001. p. 193–204.
59. Farrar EL 3rd, Lippert FG 3rd. Avulsion of the triceps tendon. Clin Orthop Relat Res 1981;161:242–6.
60. Lee ML. Rupture of the triceps tendon. Br Med J 1960;2:197.
61. Sanchez-Sotelo J, Morrey BF. Surgical techniques for reconstruction of chronic insufficiency of the triceps: rotation flap using anconeus and tendo Achilles allograft. J Bone Joint Surg Br 2002;84:1116–20.
62. Weistroffer JK, Mills WJ, Shin AY. Recurrent rupture of the triceps tendon repaired with hamstring tendon autograft augmentation: a case report and repair technique. J Shoulder Elbow Surg 2003;12:193–6.
63. Morrey BF. Radial head fractures. In: Morrey BF, editor. The elbow. Hagerstown (MD): Lippincott William & Wilkins; 2001. p. 83–102.
64. Levy M, Goldberg I, Meir I. Fracture of the head of the radius with a tear or avulsion of the triceps tendon. A new syndrome? J Bone Joint Surg Br 1982;64(1): 70–2.
65. Childress HM. Recurrent ulnar-nerve dislocation at the elbow. Clin Orthop Relat Res 1975;108:168–73.
66. Spinner RJ, Goldner RD. Snapping of the medial head of the triceps and recurrent dislocation of the ulnar nerve. Anatomical and dynamic factors. J Bone Joint Surg Am 1998;80(2):239–47.
67. Rolfsen L. Snapping triceps tendon with ulnar neuritis. Report on a case. Acta Orthop Scand 1970;41(1):74–6.

Epicondylitis in the Athlete's Elbow

Christopher Van Hofwegen, MD[a,b], Champ L. Baker III, MD[a,c],
Champ L. Baker Jr, MD[a,c,d],*

KEYWORDS

• Epicondylitis • Treatment • Postoperative care

In *Lancet* in 1882, Morris described epicondylitis in athletes and called it "lawn tennis arm."[1] The term "lawn tennis elbow" is attributed to Major[2] in an 1883 article in the *British Medical Journal*. Since then, racquet sport athletes of all kinds have been noted to be particularly susceptible to the development of lateral epicondylitis. Golfers and athletes involved in overhead throwing show a propensity to develop medial epicondylitis. In this article, both lateral and medial epicondylitis in the athlete are reviewed including pathology, clinical presentation, treatment (both nonoperative and operative) and the results of treatment are briefly reviewed.

LATERAL EPICONDYLITIS

Although lateral epicondylitis is commonly known as tennis elbow, the term is a misnomer because the condition is most often work-related and occurs in patients who do not play tennis[3]; however, it has been estimated that 10% to 50% of people who regularly play tennis do develop the condition at some time during their careers.[4] In tennis players, male players are more often affected than female players in contrast to the general population where the incidence is equal among men and women. Lateral epicondylitis occurs more frequently than medial-sided elbow pain with ratios reportedly ranging from 4:1 to 7:1.[5–7] The disorder commonly occurs in the dominant extremity. Acute onset of symptoms occurs more often in young athletes; chronic recalcitrant symptoms typically occur in older patients.

Causes

Biomechanical analysis has shown that eccentric contractions of the extensor carpi radialis brevis (ECRB) muscle during backhand tennis swings, especially in novice

---

a The Hughston Foundation, Columbus, GA, USA
b Pacific Rim Orthopaedics, 2979 Squalicum Parkway Suite 203, Bellingham, WA 98225, USA
c The Hughston Clinic, 6262 Veterans Parkway, PO Box 9517, Columbus, GA 31908, USA
d Department of Orthopaedic Surgery, Medical College of Georgia, Augusta, GA 30912, USA
* Corresponding author. The Hughston Clinic, PC, 6262 Veterans Parkway, PO Box 9517, Columbus, GA 31908-9517.
E-mail address: clbaker@hughston.com

Clin Sports Med 29 (2010) 577–597
doi:10.1016/j.csm.2010.06.009
0278-5919/10/$ – see front matter © 2010 Elsevier Inc. All rights reserved.

players, are the cause of repetitive microtrauma that results in tears to the origin of the tendon and resultant lateral epicondylitis (**Fig. 1**).[8] Some other suggested causes of lateral epicondylitis are direct trauma to the lateral region of the elbow, relative hypovascularity of the region,[9] fluoroquinolone antibiotics,[10] and anatomic predisposition.[11]

Although the term epicondylitis implies that inflammation is present, it is only present at the very early stages of the disease. Researchers have come to prefer the term tendinosis, which is defined by vascular hyperplasia and active fibroblasts.[12,13] In 1936, Cyriax[14] postulated that microscopic or macroscopic tears of the common extensor origin were involved in the disease process. Subsequently, other investigators showed that the disease process is actually a degenerative tendinopathy. Goldie[15] described granulation tissue found at the origin of the ECRB. Coonrad and Hooper[3] were the first to describe macroscopic tearing in association with the histologic findings. Nirschl[4,16] termed these histologic findings "angiofibroblastic hyperplasia." The term has since been modified to angiofibroblastic tendinosis. He noted that the gray friable tissue was characterized by disorganized, immature collagen formation with immature fibroblastic and vascular elements. Subsequently, increased rates of apoptosis and cellular autophagy have been observed in tenocytes, resulting in disruption of extracellular collagen matrix and weakening of the tendon.[17]

Regan and colleagues[18] examined the histopathologic features of 11 patients with lateral epicondylitis and confirmed that the cause of recalcitrant lateral epicondylitis indicated a degenerative rather than an inflammatory process. These changes found in the origin are the pathologic healing response to microtears caused by repetitive eccentric or concentric overloading of the extensor muscle mass.[19] Although the base of the ECRB is always involved, several studies have suggested that the origin of the extensor digitorum communis (EDC) is also implicated in lateral epicondylitis.[20,21]

Clinical Presentation

Patients who have lateral epicondylitis present with pain at the lateral aspect of the elbow that often radiates down the forearm. Occasionally, the patient can recall a specific injury to the area, but often the pain is of gradual, insidious onset, further

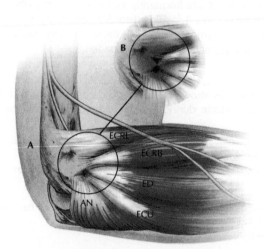

Fig. 1. (A) Normal anatomy and (B) location of pathologic tendinosis at the ECRB origin. FCR, flexor carpi radialis; FCU, flexor carpi ulnaris; PL, palmaris longus; PT, pronator teres; PUCL, posterior bundle ulnar collateral ligament; UN, ulnar nerve.

supporting its characterization as an overuse injury. They often report weakness in their grip strength or difficulty carrying items in their hand.

The physical examination portion of the evaluation for lateral epicondylitis should begin with the cervical spine and be followed by the entire upper extremity. A thorough shoulder examination is important because some patients have tight posterior capsules that may contribute to elbow pain.

The examination then proceeds to the elbow. In lateral epicondylitis, the elbow is tender over the lateral epicondyle and slightly distally into the extensor mass. Pain can be exacerbated by resisted wrist extension with the elbow in full extension and forearm in pronation (Thomsen maneuver) or by maximal wrist flexion. The first maneuver causes painful eccentric contraction at the origin of the ECRB. The second maneuver places the ECRB on maximal stretch, passively tensioning the muscle origin causing pain. Testing for a plica involves passively flexing the elbow with the forearm pronated and supinated. Plica can be differentiated from lateral epicondylitis by the point of maximal tenderness, which is located more distally and posteriorly over the radiocapitellar joint. Radial tunnel syndrome and posterior interosseous nerve (PIN) syndrome are nerve entrapments at 1 or more sites resulting in pain on the lateral side of the arm. In as many as 5% of patients with lateral epicondylitis, radial nerve entrapment occurs simultaneously.[22] Pain on resisted supination (when the nerve is trapped in the supinator muscle) or pain with resisted long-finger extension (when the nerve is trapped in the ECRB) can indicate radial nerve entrapment. Distinguishing between nerve entrapment on the lateral side of the arm and lateral epicondylitis can be difficult. It is important to do so, however, because treatment of the 2 conditions is entirely different. The elbow examination is completed with a standard evaluation of elbow stability, range of motion, and effusion.

The examination moves distally into the forearm and hand. Grip strength should be tested to determine whether it is decreased compared with the unaffected side or causes significant discomfort. Neurovascular status is a basic component of the examination and should be noted.

The differential diagnosis for lateral elbow pain includes synovial plica, osteochondritis dissecans of the capitellum, radiocapitellar arthrosis, radial tunnel syndrome, cervical radiculopathy, and posterolateral rotatory instability.

Although they are usually ordered in the clinical setting, imaging studies are usually more helpful in excluding other causes of lateral elbow pain than in making the diagnosis of lateral epicondylitis. Radiography can demonstrate calcifications in the soft tissues around the lateral epicondyle in about one-quarter of patients with the condition (Fig. 2).[23] Magnetic resonance imaging (MRI), although not generally indicated, is useful in the exclusion of intraarticular pathology such as osteochondral defects and chondral loose bodies, as well as more subtle findings such as nondisplaced physeal fractures. When MRI is used to image lateral epicondylitis, the imaging findings of tendon degeneration and degree of the tear correlate well with surgical and histologic findings.[19] T1- and T2-weighted images show increased signal around the lateral epicondyle, which corresponds to mucoid degeneration and neovascularization. Coel and colleagues[24] noted increased MRI signal changes in the anconeus muscle in patients with recalcitrant lateral epicondylitis, but were not able to determine whether this increased signal was associated with chronicity of the symptoms or with abnormal elbow motion as a result of the patient's symptoms.

Nonoperative Treatment

The success rate of nonoperative treatment can be up to 90%.[14,25–41] It includes patient education, physical therapy, medications, acupuncture, braces,

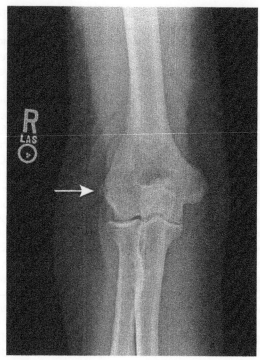

Fig. 2. Anteroposterior radiograph of the elbow demonstrating abnormal lateral calcification.

extracorporeal shock wave therapy (ESWT), iontophoresis, and injections. Cessation of the offending activity, or active rest is critical to success. The first step in achieving that is with patient education, including a frank discussion of the pathoanatomy and ways to avoid aggravating activities. If the epicondylitis occurs in a tennis player and can be attributed to the sport, special attention should be always paid to proper technique. It is important that the grip of the tennis racket be checked for proper sizing, and the weight and the string tension of the racket be checked as possible causes of the problem.

Physical therapy can include such modalities as friction massage,[14] manipulation,[26] and stretching and strengthening the extensor wad when the pain subsides. In combination with oral analgesics, therapy can be effective. Our therapy program consists of oral nonsteroidal antiinflammatory medications, rest, activity modification, strengthening exercises, and counterforce bracing (**Box 1**).[42] Other therapy modalities can include cryotherapy, electrical stimulation, ultrasound,[27] and iontophoresis.[28] Medications include acetaminophen and a variety of oral or topical nonsteroidal antiinflammatory medications.[29]

Counterforce or wrist extension braces can be helpful. The counterforce brace, introduced in the early 1970s, is believed to reduce the load at the lateral epicondyle by preventing the forearm muscles from fully expanding. Although there are several types of braces on the market, Walther and colleagues[36] showed that any brace that placed a compressive pad just distal to the lateral epicondyle resulted in a higher reduction of load at the lateral epicondyle than braces using the principle of a clasp, and braces placed just distal to the lateral epicondyle reduced loads greater than

---

Box 1
Nonoperative treatment protocol for lateral epicondylitis

Initial treatment

Reduce pain, inflammation, edema

Rest from aggravating activities

Antiinflammatory medication, phonophoresis, iontophoresis

Deep friction massage (2–3 minutes, 2 times a day)

Ice massage (5 minutes, 2 times a day)

Stretching (30 seconds for 5 repetitions, 3 times a day):

- Elbow flexion/extension
- Wrist flexion/extension
- Forearm pronation/supination

Grip strengthening (2–3 minutes, 2 times a day)

Counterforce bracing

Intermediate phase

Continue stretching, appropriate modalities, and bracing

Initiate progressive pain-free resistive strengthening (3 sets of 15, 2 times a day)

- Wrist curls (0–0.9 kg [0–2 lb] progressing to 1.3–2.2 kg [3–5 lb])
- Elbow flexion/extension (0.9–1.3 kg [2–3 lb] progressing to 2.2–4.5 kg [5–10 lb])
- Forearm pronation/supination (0–0.9 kg [0–2 lb] progressing to 1.3–2.2 kg [3–5 lb])

Shoulder strengthening to prevent disuse atrophy

Resume previously aggravating activities

Final phase of rehabilitation

Continue stretching and strengthening

Functional training, correct mechanics

Ice after activity

Gradual return to sport

Maintenance stretching and strengthening program 3 times a week

---

pads placed over the lateral epicondyle. The wrist extension brace places the arm in a position of rest for the extensors.

ESWT, the vibration of shock waves through tissue, is believed to activate the cycle of inflammation in the hope that it will complete its course to resolution of symptoms. There has been contradicting evidence as to the efficacy of ESWT. Some investigators noted that patients who received ESWT had improved symptoms.[37–39] Other studies, however, have reported a lack of effectiveness with ESWT.[33–38,40] Side effects from this treatment include transient reddening of the skin, pain at the site of the treatment, small hematomas, migraines, and syncope.[41]

Injections of a local anesthetic and a corticosteroid are often helpful. However, conflicting data have been published regarding the long-term efficacy of injections. Altay and colleagues[30] reported that injecting lidocaine and triamcinolone in a peppering technique was reliable in treating this disease. Others reported that the beneficial effect of the injections is only transient.[31] Newcomer and colleagues[32] questioned the results of corticosteroid injections in relieving the early (<4 weeks) symptoms of lateral epicondylitis and found that they did not help significantly. Crowther and colleagues[33] noted that, compared with ESWT, the steroid injections worked better and were less expensive at 3 months. At 6 weeks follow-up, Verhaar and colleagues[34] found steroid injections to be more beneficial than manipulation using the Cyriax method. Judicious use of injections is important to avoid known possible side effects of skin discolorations and fat atrophy at the site of the injection.

Other types of injections include botulinum toxin injection. Placzek and colleagues[43] compared botulinum toxin A injections with placebo in a prospective randomized, controlled, double-blind trial. Their results showed botulinum toxin to be statistically superior to placebo for relief of and resolution of symptoms. Keizer and colleagues[35] performed a prospective study to compare the results of open surgical treatment and injection with botulinum toxin. One year after treatment, 65% of their patients injected with botulinum and 75% of patients treated surgically had good to excellent results. At 2 years after treatment, the success rate for the injection cohort increased to 75%.

The use of platelet-rich plasma (PRP) has also been investigated to a limited extent for its use in treatment of lateral epicondylitis.[44,45] PRP has been documented to release massive quantities of advantageous cytokines such as vascular endothelial growth factor and platelet-derived growth factor known to be important in tendon healing.[44,45] Peerbooms and colleagues[44] published a randomized controlled trial comparing the effects of PRP injections with steroid injections for lateral epicondylitis and found that at 1 year, patients injected with PRP had significantly improved pain and functional scores compared with those who were injected with steroids. The investigators concluded that it was an effective treatment but also suggested that more studies should be done not only to confirm their findings but also to decipher the mechanism of action and risk profile for the treatment.

Mishra and Pavelko[45] reported on the use of PRP injections on patients with recalcitrant lateral epicondylitis who had otherwise exhausted common conservative measures. The investigators injected bupivacaine in the control group or PRP in the experimental group at the sight of the common extensor origin. At 8 weeks, the bupivacaine group experienced 16% relief of pain, whereas the PRP group experienced 60% relief. Unfortunately, at this point in the study, 60% of the control group dropped out and sought other treatment, so the final analysis was limited to the experimental group. However, the final analysis was impressive with patients injected with PRP reporting 93% relief of pain at slightly more than 2 years.

The effects of whole-blood injections have also been studied. Connell and colleagues[46] used ultrasound guidance to place injections and subsequent ultrasounds to monitor changes at the sight of the injections. The investigators also monitored pain relief using the Nirschl criteria and visual analog scores (VAS). They concluded that although there was continued ultrasonic evidence of abnormality within the extensor origin, patients' symptoms improved on the Nirschl scale from an average of 6 to 0 and on the VAS from 9 to 0 at 6 months. Unfortunately, the study was uncontrolled. Ul Gani and colleagues[47] reported less optimistic results. They showed significant improvement in pain and Nirschl staging in 58% of patients who received autologous blood injections, leaving 42% of patients with an unsatisfactory response.

Prolotherapy is the practice of injecting an irritant substance (eg, hyperosmolar dextrose, sodium morrhuate) into a ligament or tendon to promote the growth of new tissue. Its use has been documented as far back as the 1930s, when it was used for pain presumed to originate from tissue laxity.[48] Although tissue laxity is not the impetus for use in lateral epicondylitis, the practice has been modernized and evaluated in recent times regarding its efficacy. Scarpone and colleagues[49] performed a double-blinded, randomized, controlled trial to evaluate the technique and assessed both pain relief and function objectively at 8 and 16 weeks after intervention. Their results showed injection of sodium morrhuate to be statistically significantly better for relief of pain and improvement of function compared with controls.

As an alternative to hypodermic administration, iontophoresis, or the use of electrical current as a delivery mechanism for steroids, has also been studied. Nirschl[16] studied the use of iontophoresis for treatment in acute medial and lateral epicondylitis. The study group noted significant improvement in pain scores compared with the placebo group in the first several days. However, the difference in pain improvement was not maintained at 1 month. Both groups noted overall improvement.

Nitric oxide has been reported to be an important factor in tendon healing. Animal studies and cell culture support the theory that nitric oxide enhances extracellular matrix production, improving mechanical properties.[50] Paoloni and colleagues[51] described the clinical use of nitric oxide with lateral epicondylitis by performing a prospective, randomized, double-blinded clinical trial. The investigators compared equivalent cohorts of patients receiving standard rehabilitation and nitroglycerine patches or rehabilitation and placebo patches. Patients in the nitroglycerine group had significantly reduced elbow pain with activity at 2 weeks and reduced epicondylar tenderness at 6 and 12 weeks. Patients receiving nitroglycerine patches also showed increased wrist extensor strength at 24 weeks. At 6 months, 81% of treated patients were asymptomatic during activities of daily living, compared with 60% of patients who had tendon rehabilitation alone. The investigators concluded that topical nitroglycerine patches were effective in the treatment of lateral epicondylitis.

Operative Treatment

Most patients respond successfully to the variety of conservative treatment methods previously discussed. According to the reports of large patient series by Nirschl and Pettrone,[52] Boyd and McLeod,[53] and Coonrad and Hooper,[3] 4% to 11% of patients ultimately require operative intervention for recalcitrant symptoms. Surgical treatment is indicated for those patients with continued symptoms and disability despite appropriate nonoperative management. Many different operative procedures for the treatment of lateral epicondylitis have been described in the literature including a percutaneous,[54–59] endoscopic,[60,61] or open release of the common extensor tendon origin[61–64]; an extensor release with additional intraarticular modifications[45,65]; an extensor fasciotomy[66]; a V-Y slide of the common extensor origin[67]; denervation of the lateral epicondyle[68,69]; epicondylar resection with aconeus muscle transfer[70]; distal lengthening of the ECRB at the wrist[71–73]; extensor tendon repair and advancement[74]; excision of the abnormal degenerative tissue with simple suture repair[3,52,55,58,75–78]; and excision of the abnormal degenerative tissue with formal repair of the extensor tendons back to the lateral epicondyle.[1,79,80] More recently, arthroscopic techniques in the management of lateral epicondylitis have been reported.[58,76,81–89]

Regardless of the technique chosen, successful operative treatment of lateral epicondylitis is primarily dependent on proper patient selection, identification of pathology, and complete resection of the ECRB tendinosis. The ECRB angiofibroblastic tendinosis tissue can be easily resected via an open or arthroscopic approach. In the open technique as popularized by Nirschl and associates,[13,52,78] the patient is positioned supine on the operating table with an attached arm board. With the affected extremity under tourniquet control, a 4-cm incision is made anteromedial to the lateral epicondyle (**Fig. 3**). The subcutaneous tissues are divided to the level of the deep fascia overlying the extensor tendons. The interface between the extensor carpi radialis longus (ECRL) anteriorly and EDC aponeurosis posteriorly is identified and split superficially to a depth of 2 to 3 mm. The ECRL is then separated from the underlying ECRB by scalpel dissection and retracted anteriorly. The pathologic ECRB tissue is now readily identified by its dull, gray appearance. All abnormal tissue is excised sharply en bloc (**Fig. 4**). Vascular supply is enhanced with drilling of the lateral condyle. The ECRL and EDC aponeurosis are reapproximated with a running no. 1 absorbable suture. Next, the subcutaneous tissues and skin are closed in routine fashion. A posterior split is applied with the elbow in 90° of flexion for 1 week to allow for wound healing. Range-of-motion exercises for the elbow and wrist are instituted and are followed by strengthening when the patient has attained full painless motion. Return to sports is allowed as tolerated, typically at 6 to 8 weeks after surgery.

Open resection of tendinosis tissue provides a high rate of successful outcomes and return to sport at both short- and long-term follow-up.[52,78] In a large series of 92 elbows in 83 patients, at an average follow-up of 12.6 years, 84% of patients had good or excellent outcomes based on the Nirschl tennis elbow score and Verhaar criteria.[64] Ninety-seven percent of patients were improved, and 93% of athletes were able to return to sporting activities.

Alternatively, arthroscopic release of the ECRB origin with resection of the pathologic tendinosis tissue provides reproducible pain relief and potentially allows patients to return to unrestricted activities sooner than open surgery. Cadaveric studies have demonstrated the ability to completely resect the entire ECRB origin safely without violation of the important lateral ligamentous complex.[90–92] The arthroscopic technique also allows for the identification and treatment of coexistent intraarticular pathology. Our preference is to perform elbow arthroscopy with the patient prone under general anesthesia. A nonsterile tourniquet is applied with the affected extremity in an arm holder. After distention of the elbow joint with normal saline introduced through the soft spot lateral portal, a proximal anteromedial portal is created first for joint inspection. The lateral capsule is evaluated for capsular tears, synovial

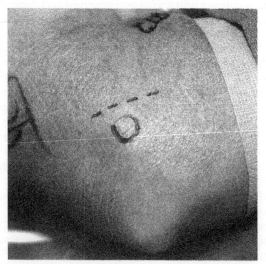

Fig. 3. A limited approach for open resection is made just anteromedial to the marked lateral epicondyle.

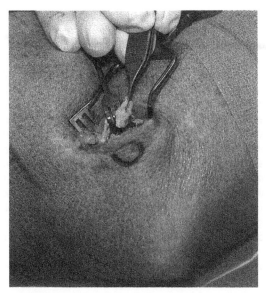

Fig. 4. The abnormal tendinosis tissue is resected en bloc.

thickening, or extension of the annular ligament overlying the radial head (**Fig. 5**). Radiocapitellar chondromalacia may also been seen. A proximal anterolateral portal is created under direct visualization. A shaver is introduced through this portal and a portion of the lateral capsule is resected to reveal the common extensor tendon. The ECRB tendon lies between the common extensor origin and the removed capsule. The shaver is exchanged for a monopolar radiofrequency device. The tendinosis tissue is ablated with complete resection of the ECRB origin off the lateral humerus. Care is taken not to extend the resection posterior to a line bisecting the radial head to protect the lateral ligamentous structures. Portal sites are closed routinely and a sterile soft dressing applied. Patients are encouraged to initiate active and passive range-of-motion exercises immediately. If the patient has difficulty regaining full extension by the end of the first week then formal physical therapy is prescribed. Otherwise, as patient symptoms allow simple stretching and strengthening exercises

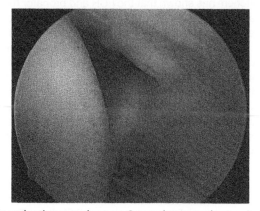

Fig. 5. Arthroscopic evaluation reveals a type 3 complete capsular tear in the left elbow with the patient in the prone position. View is from the proximal medial portal.

are initiated. Patients typically return to light activities at 2 weeks after surgery and to sports at approximately 6 weeks.

Short-term results after arthroscopic treatment of lateral epicondylitis have high rates of success with pain relief and return to activities.[58,76,81,84–86,88,89] The authors recently performed a long-term follow-up study of 30 elbows in 30 patients treated with arthroscopic resection of the ECRB origin for lateral epicondylitis.[82] At a mean follow-up of 130 months, the mean pain score at rest was 0; for activities of daily living, the mean score was 1.0; and for work or sports, the mean score was 1.9 out of 10. The mean functional score was 11.7 out of a possible 12 points on the Mayo Clinic Elbow Performance Index. No patient required repeat injections or surgeries. Eighty-seven percent of patients were satisfied, and 97% of patients stated they were "much better" or "better" at final follow-up. In a comparative retrospective study, Szabo and colleagues[58] evaluated 23 percutaneous, 38 open, and 41 arthroscopic procedures at a mean follow-up of 48 months. There were no statistically significant differences among the 3 surgical groups with regard to recurrences, complications, failures, preoperative or postoperative Andrews-Carson scores, or visual analog pain scores. The investigators were unable to determine the rate at which the patients returned to work and activities of daily living without discomfort, but they concluded that each method is a highly effective way to treat recalcitrant lateral epicondylitis.

MEDIAL EPICONDYLITIS
Causes

Medial epicondylitis, often called golfer's elbow, can affect all athletes who repetitively contract the flexor-pronator mass. Medial epicondylitis results from the pathologic combination of intrinsic muscle contraction of the flexor-pronator muscles added to the extrinsic valgus force of swinging or throwing. Athletes who have been noted to be particularly susceptible to the development of medial epicondylitis are golfers and athletes involved in overhead throwing. Medial epicondylitis has been noted in athletes of many different sports including bowling, racquetball, football, archery, weightlifting, and javelin throwing.[93] Much like lateral epicondylitis, this condition is not limited to the athletic population but is also associated with many occupations in which repetitive wrist flexion and pronation are required, such as carpentry.

The flexor carpi radialis (FCR) and pronator teres have been the most consistently implicated sites for development of medial epicondylitis (**Fig. 6**). Electromyographic (EMG) analysis of pitchers has shown that the FCR and pronator teres are most active during the acceleration phase of a pitch.[94] When this is coupled with the extreme valgus torque forces producing acceleration of as much as 600,000 degrees/s^2,[95] significant tension is placed in the origin of the flexor mass. Repetitive exposure of the medial aspect of the elbow to this combined force in the context of bad mechanics, inadequate warm up, poor conditioning, or overuse can overcome the tensile strength of the muscles' origins, causing microtearing. The persistent tension over the microtears at the origin of the FCR and pronator teres causes the pathologic healing response termed angiofibroblastic tendinosis. Similar to lateral epicondylitis, medial epicondylitis is characterized by disorganized, immature collagen formation with immature fibroblastic and vascular elements.

Anatomy

The anatomy of the medial aspect of the elbow must be kept in mind when considering a diagnosis of medial epicondylitis, as it can be difficult to distinguish from other causes of medial elbow pain. In general, medial elbow pain is a common complaint

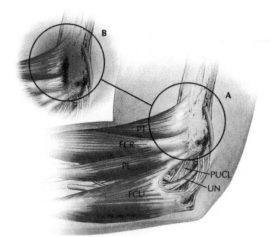

Fig. 6. (A) Normal anatomy and (B) the typical location of pathology at the FCR-palmaris longus origin. AN, anconeus; ECRB, extensor carpi radialis brevis; ECRL, extensor carpi radialis longus; ECU, extensor carpi ulnaris; ED, extensor digitorum.

in athletes involved in overhead throwing, accounting for 97% of elbow complaints in pitchers.[95] Other causes of medial elbow pain include ulnar collateral ligament injury, ulnar neuropraxia, or medial elbow intraarticular pathology.[22] The diagnosis is especially difficult because diagnosis of 1 pathologic entity does not preclude, but more often includes, another diagnosis. Ulnar neuritis has been reported with medial epicondylitis approximately 60% of the time.[22] Conway and colleagues[96] reported on outcomes of athletes involved in overhead throwing who had undergone ulnar collateral ligament reconstruction versus repair and noted nearly 15% of them had undiagnosed muscle belly ruptures of the flexor-pronator mass. These reports highlight the probability of coincident pathology in a single elbow, making keen recall of the anatomy of paramount importance during the physical examination.

The anatomy of the medial elbow from deep to superficial begins with the osseous articulation of the ulna and humerus. Bony anatomy is believed to provide valgus stability to the elbow in up to 20° of flexion and beyond 120° of flexion. Soft tissue provides the primary restraint to valgus load from 20° to 120° of flexion.[97]

The primary soft tissue restraint on the medial aspect of the elbow is the ulnar collateral ligament, which is divided into 3 bundles: anterior, posterior, and transverse. The anterior band of the ulnar collateral ligament is the most important structure in resisting valgus load and can be further divided into anterior and posterior bands.[98] These bands are functional at slightly different times: anterior up to 90° and posterior from 60° to full flexion.

Passing through the cubital tunnel superficial to the ulnar collateral ligament is the ulnar nerve. As it enters the tunnel, the ulnar nerve courses posterior to the medial intermuscular septum and the medial epicondyle. In the tunnel, it is located directly superficial to the ulnar collateral ligament and deep to the Osborne ligament. The nerve then travels distally between the 2 heads of the flexor carpi ulnaris (FCU) of the flexor-pronator muscle mass. Ollivierre and colleagues[99] divided the course of the ulnar nerve into 3 zones. The first zone is proximal to the medial epicondyle, the second is at the medial epicondyle, and the third is distal to the medial epicondyle. They found the third zone to be the most common site of ulnar nerve compression as the nerve enters the FCU arcade. This finding was established in patients who were undergoing surgical debridement for medial epicondylitis and had concomitant ulnar nerve compression.

The flexor-pronator muscles originate from the medial epicondyle and include the pronator teres, FCR, palmaris longus, flexor digitorum superficialis (FDS), and FCU. The FCU has both humeral and ulnar heads. The pronator teres and FCR are anatomic structures most commonly involved in medial epicondylitis, and they originate from the medial supracondylar ridge.[1]

Clinical Presentation

Patients who have medial epicondylitis tend to report a gradual onset and increase of medial symptoms without a particular inciting event. Pain is usually noted during the acceleration phase of throwing when the FCR and pronator teres are most active. Pain localizes to either the medial epicondyle or just distal in the flexor-pronator mass. However, as discussed earlier, pain over the flexor-pronator mass is not necessarily specific to medial epicondylitis, and its presence necessitates a complete elbow examination and evaluation of the deeper structures.

A differential diagnosis generated from the history guides the physical examination. The differential for medial elbow pain includes medial epicondylitis, ulnar neuritis, ulnar collateral ligament attenuation with resultant instability, or flexor pronator muscle belly ruptures. Depending on the patient's age, Little League elbow, or physeal fracture of the medial epicondyle, can also be suspected. Older athletes tend to have insidious onset of symptoms unless there is an acute muscle belly rupture.

Pain from medial epicondylitis most often can be elicited on examination by palpating the medial epicondyle and slightly distally into the flexor pronator mass. However, tenderness in the flexor-pronator mass is not necessarily specific to epicondylitis and can also be present in ulnar collateral ligament instability or ulnar neuritis. Pain during resisted pronation has been reported to be the most sensitive physical examination finding.[100] Pain during resisted wrist flexion can also indicate medial epicondylitis.

Ulnar neuritis can be differentiated from other causes of elbow pain by its neurologic findings. It leads to pain coupled with sensory dysesthesias into the small and ring fingers at least transiently during valgus stress of the elbow. Tinel sign is usually positive at the elbow over the course of the ulnar nerve and produces transient electrical or shocking sensations distally into the ring and small fingers. Elbow flexion testing (maximum elbow flexion, forearm in pronation, wrist in extension) often brings on gradual symptoms of ulnar nerve dysesthesias as well. Sensory testing should include 2-point discrimination, particularly in the ring and small fingers. Motor testing should include assessment of intrinsic muscles to the hand, which can be weak or atrophic. Froment sign (compensatory use of the flexor pollicis longus in contrast to the adductor pollicis when holding an object) can be positive in chronic cases. EMG studies can help to confirm the diagnosis and differentiate from proximal or distal sites of nerve compression.

Medial ulnar collateral ligament instability must also be suspected when medial elbow pain is present. The standard physical examination maneuver to diagnosis this condition involves passive valgus stress of the elbow between 20° and 90° of flexion when the anterior band of the ulnar collateral ligament is under most stress. This is often referred to as the milking maneuver. Tenderness can also be elicited with direct palpation over the ligament but is a nonspecific finding.

Avulsions of the flexor-pronator muscle belly have been documented as an acute cause of medial elbow pain,[101,102] but these injuries almost always occur in conjunction with traumatic rupture of the ulnar collateral ligament. Physical examination usually reveals pain over the flexor mass coupled with instability. In general, the finding of pain in the flexor-pronator mass is nonspecific, and advanced imaging studies, such as MRI, are a useful adjunct to making a diagnosis in this setting.

When medial epicondylitis is suspected, radiographs are used not so much for its diagnosis as for the detection of concomitant disorders. Standard radiographs of the elbow are most often normal, but they can show calcifications around the medial epicondyle (**Fig. 7**). MRI or bone scans may be necessary to determine a nondisplaced fracture of the medial epicondyle. MRI of an elbow with medial epicondylitis usually shows a thickening of the common flexor tendon origin with increased signal intensity on T1- and T2-weighted images consistent with the underlying pathoanatomy. Conversely, some individuals have areas of thinning in the common flexor tendon origin with intense fluid signals in T2-weighted images (**Fig. 8**).[19]

Nonoperative Treatment

Treatment of medial epicondylar pathology depends much on the age of the player and his or her particular circumstances. The protocol of rest, ice, and nonsteroidal antiinflammatory medication is believed to be useful for relief of epicondylitis symptoms in about 90% of patients.[100] Nonsurgical treatment is usually successful and remains the mainstay of treatment. Surgical treatment of medial epicondylitis is reserved for those patients who do not show significant improvement with rest and a supervised course of prolonged rehabilitation; a period of 6 to 12 months has been recommended.[1]

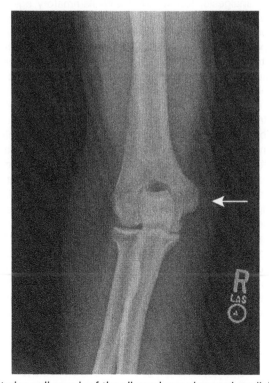

Fig. 7. Anteroposterior radiograph of the elbow shows abnormal medial calcification.

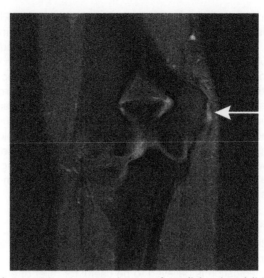

Fig. 8. T2 coronal magnetic resonance image of medial epicondylitis with pathologic increase in signal intensity at the origin of the flexor-pronator mass.

Nonoperative treatment is divided into 3 different phases. Phase 1 involves immediate and complete cessation of the offending activity, which is not to be confused with complete immobilization. The goal of phase 1 is relief of pain. Acetaminophen is a good first-line analgesic. Nonsteroidal antiinflammatory agents are also good for analgesia; however, medial epicondylitis is not a true inflammatory condition so the antiinflammatory benefits at the cellular-cytokine level are questionable. Their antiinflammatory properties may be beneficial for concomitant conditions, especially if there is an intraarticular synovitis from joint instability. Counterforce bracing may be efficacious in some patients, but it can exacerbate compressive neuropathies.

The use of steroids to treat medial epicondylitis has good results in the short-term, but significant long-term improvements have not been sustained compared with conservative treatment alone. In a prospective study of steroid injections for medial epicondylitis, patients who received steroid injections reported significantly improved pain scores and more rapid improvement in their symptoms compared with those in control patients at 6 weeks.[103] These results were not maintained at 3-month and 1-year follow-up examinations. Aside from not maintaining their benefits, medial epicondylar injections have known associated complications including attenuation of medial collateral ligament from direct inoculation, chemical neuritis,[104] skin atrophy, and pigment changes.

As an alternative to hypodermic administration, iontophoresis, or the use of electrical current as a delivery mechanism for steroids, has also been studied. Nirschl and colleagues[28] studied the use of iontophoresis for treatment in acute medial and lateral epicondylitis. The study group noted significant improvement in pain scores compared with the placebo group in the first several days. However, the difference in pain improvement was not maintained at 1 month. Both groups noted overall improvement.

When symptoms have resolved, phase 2 of rehabilitation is initiated. The goal of phase 2 is to regain range of motion of the elbow and wrist and then to increase strength. This phase usually involves guided physical therapy, begun with little, if any, resistance, that is gradually increased in intensity and duration. When symptom-free range of motion has been achieved and strengthening is optimized, the athlete moves on to phase 3, which is returning to sport. This phase involves correction of the underlying cause, such as poor technique, equipment issues, or lack of conditioning, which is imperative in maintaining symptom relief.

Operative Treatment

The primary indication for surgical treatment of medial epicondylitis is persistent pain and disability despite an appropriate course of nonoperative management of at least 6 months in duration. In contrast to the myriad of operative techniques described for lateral epicondylitis, there are few published reports describing the operative management of medial epicondylitis. Surgical options include percutaneous epicondylar muscle release,[54] open detachment of the flexor muscle origin without debridement,[105] open detachment of the flexor origin with debridement of pathologic tendinosis tissue followed by secure common flexor repair,[1,106] open medial epicondylectomy, and open resection of pathologic tendinosis tissue.[99]

Our preferred operative technique is similar to that described by Olivierre and colleagues.[99] The patient is evaluated in the preoperative holding area, and the point of maximal tenderness is marked. The patient is then positioned supine on the operating table with the affected extremity placed on an attached arm board. General anesthesia and prophylactic intravenous antibiotics are administered. A well-padded tourniquet is placed proximally about the brachium. The upper extremity is sterilely prepared and draped and the limb is exsanguinated. A slightly curvilinear incision is made starting approximately 2 cm proximal and extending 4 cm distal to the medial epicondyle. This incision parallels the epicondylar groove and is placed posterior to the epicondyle to avoid iatrogenic injury to the medial antebrachial cutaneous nerve and to provide concurrent complete access to the ulnar nerve, if needed. Dissection proceeds through the subcutaneous tissues until the deep fascia of the FCU is identified. Further dissection proceeds anterolaterally in this plane to expose the common flexor origin.

A longitudinal incision is made in the common flexor origin overlying the point of maximal tenderness starting at the medial epicondyle and extending distally approximately 4 cm. The incision is typically located in the interval between the pronator teres and FCR. The pathologic tendinosis tissue is readily exposed as the interval is deepened. The dull, gray abnormal tissue is identified and separated from healthy tendon. Total excision of all pathologic tissue is performed in an elliptical fashion. The scratch maneuver as described by Ollivierre and colleagues[99] may help to identify abnormal tissue to be excised.

Careful preoperative evaluation regarding the presence and severity of ulnar nerve symptoms dictate intraoperative management. Ulnar nerve involvement has been variously reported in 23% to 60% of patients requiring operative intervention.[99,100,105,106] Gabel and Morrey[100] noted the influence of concurrent ulnar neuropathy and its effect on outcome when preoperative symptoms are moderate to severe. In patients with mild ulnar nerve symptoms preoperatively, we prefer to perform an in situ ulnar nerve decompression. We reserve an anterior subcutaneous ulnar nerve transposition for those cases with preoperative moderate or severe ulnar neuropathy or with evidence of a subluxating or dislocating ulnar nerve as the elbow is brought into full range of motion.

Multiple holes are drilled in the cortical bone just distal to the medial epicondyle with a 0.062 Kirschner wire to stimulate a healing response. The elliptical tendon defect is closed with a no. 1 absorbable suture followed by subcutaneous layer closure. The skin is closed with a running subcuticular stitch with 3-0 absorbable suture. A posterior splint is applied with the elbow in approximately 90° of flexion and neutral rotation.

The splint is removed approximately 1 week after surgery and range-of-motion exercises for the elbow and wrist are begun. Gentle strengthening exercises are begun around 4 to 6 weeks after surgery. A counterforce brace is worn for therapy and for more vigorous activities of daily living. Once painless full motion and strength are achieved, the patient is allowed to resume full sports participation without restrictions usually at 4 to 5 months postoperatively.

Vangsness and Jobe[106] evaluated the results of 35 patients treated with common flexor origin detachment, tendinosis tissue debridement, medial epicondyle drilling, and secure common flexor repair at a mean 85 months follow-up. The investigators reported overall 97% excellent to good results with 95% of patients returning to previous level of sporting activities without limitations. Kurvers and Verhaar[105] performed open division of the common flexor origin in 40 patients. No tissue debridement was performed. At a mean follow-up of 44 months, 25 patients (63%) reported good subjective outcomes. The presence of coexistent ulnar neuritis was associated with an overall poor subjective outcome. Similarly, Gabel and Morrey[100] noted good to excellent results in 40% of elbows with concurrent moderate to severe ulnar neuropathy compared with 96% good to excellent results in elbows with no or only mild ulnar neuritis. Overall, the investigators reported 87% good to excellent results in their series of 30 elbows treated with flexor-pronator origin debridement at an average 7-year follow-up. Ollivierre and colleagues[99] evaluated the results of resection of pathologic tendinosis tissue and closure of the excision defect in 50 elbows at a mean follow-up of 37 months. All patients reported improvement in their pain. Sixty-nine percent of patients were able to return to their sporting activities.

SUMMARY

Epicondylitis in the athlete is caused by a pathologic healing response to repetitive eccentric contraction of the flexor or extensor muscles at their respective origins in the elbow. The pathologic angiofibroblastic tendinosis of lateral epicondylitis is usually found at the base of the ECRB and for the most part is an isolated entity in its presentation. Medial epicondylitis is found at the base of the FCR and pronator teres. It needs to be carefully differentiated from other causes of medial elbow pain because of its propensity for concurrent presentation with other causes of medial pain such as ulnar collateral ligament instability or ulnar neuritis.

Treatment of epicondylitis in athletes is aimed at resolution of symptoms with resumption of sport. For the most part, conservative treatment, consisting of active rest, injections, bracing, physical therapy, and correction of the underlying cause, has been successful. In recalcitrant cases, surgery for both lateral and medial epicondylitis has been suggested. For lateral epicondylitis, multiple methods including open, percutaneous, and arthroscopic techniques have been reported. Because of the proximity of the ulnar nerve, surgical reports for medial epicondylitis have been limited to open and percutaneous techniques. Regardless of the technique, pain relief is usually reliable, whereas return to sport with complete resolution of symptoms is less predictable, especially when epicondylitis presents with concomitant pathology.

REFERENCES

1. Jobe FW, Cicotti MG. Lateral and medial epicondylitis of the elbow. J Am Acad Orthop Surg 1994;2:1–8.
2. Major HP. Lawn-tennis elbow. Br Med J 1883;2:557.
3. Coonrad RW, Hooper WR. Tennis elbow: its courses, natural history, conservative and surgical management. J Bone Joint Surg Am 1973;55:1177–82.

4. Nirschl RP. Elbow tendinosis/tennis elbow. Clin Sports Med 1992;11:851–70.

5. Gabel GT, Morrey BF. Tennis elbow. Instr Course Lect 1998;47:165–72.

6. Leach RE, Miller JK. Lateral and medial epicondylitis of the elbow. Clin Sports Med 1987;6:259–72.

7. Nirschl RP. Soft-tissue injuries about the elbow. Clin Sports Med 1986;5:637–52.

8. Riek S, Chapman AE, Milner T. A simulation of muscle force and internal kinematics of extensor carpi radialis brevis during backhand tennis stroke: implications for injury. Clin Biomech 1999;14:477–83.

9. Schneeberger AG, Masquelet AC. Arterial vascularization of the proximal extensor carpi radialis brevis tendon. Clin Orthop Relat Res 2002;398:239–44.

10. LeHuec JC, Schaeverbeke T, Chauveaux D, et al. Epicondylitis after treatment with fluoroquinolone antibiotics. J Bone Joint Surg Br 1995;77:293–5.

11. Bunata RE, Brown DS, Capelo R. Anatomic factors related to the causes of tennis elbow. J Bone Joint Surg Am 2007;89:1955–63.

12. Kraushaar BS, Nirschl RP. Tendinosis of the elbow (tennis elbow). Clinical features and findings of histological, immunohistochemical, and electron microscopy studies. J Bone Joint Surg Am 1999;81:259–78.

13. Baker CL, Nirschl RP. Lateral tendon injury: open and arthroscopic treatment. In: Altchek DW, Andrews JR, editors. The athlete's elbow. Philadelphia: Lippincott Williams & Wilkins; 2001. p. 91–103.

14. Cyriax JH. The pathology and treatment of tennis elbow. J Bone Joint Surg 1936; 18:921–40.

15. Goldie I. Epicondylitis lateralis humeri (epicondylagia or tennis elbow) A pathologic study. Acta Chir Scand Suppl 1964;339.

16. Nirschl RP. Muscle and tendon trauma: tennis elbow. In: Morrey BF, editor. The elbow and its disorders. 1st edition. Philadelphia: WB Saunders; 1985. p. 537–52.

17. Chen J, Wang A, Xu J, et al. In chronic lateral epicondylitis, apoptosis and autophagic cell death occur in the extensor carpi radialis brevis tendon. J Shoulder Elbow Surg 2010;19:355–62.

18. Regan W, Wold LE, Coonrad R, et al. Microscopic histopathology of chronic refractory lateral epicondylitis. Am J Sports Med 1992;20(6):746–9.

19. Tuite MJ, Kijowski R. Sports-related injuries of the elbow: an approach to MRI interpretation. Clin Sports Med 2006;25:387–408, v.

20. Fairbank SM, Corlett RJ. The role of the extensor digitorum communis muscle in lateral epicondylitis. J Hand Surg Br 2002;27(5):405–9.

21. Greenbaum B, Itamura J, Vangsness CT, et al. Extensor carpi radialis brevis. An anatomical analysis of its origin. J Bone Joint Surg Br 1999;81:926–9.

22. Field LD, Savoie FH. Common elbow injuries in sport. Sports Med 1998;26: 193–205.

23. Edelson G, Kunos CA, Vigder F, et al. Bony changes at the lateral epicondyle of possible significance in tennis elbow syndrome. J Shoulder Elbow Surg 2001; 10(2):158–63.

24. Coel M, Yamada CY, Ko J. MR imaging of patients with lateral epicondylitis of the elbow (tennis elbow): importance of increase signal of the anconeus muscle. AJR Am J Roentgenol 1993;161:1019–21.

25. Brattberg G. Acupuncture therapy for tennis elbow. Pain 1983;16:285–8.

26. Mills GP. The treatment of tennis elbow. Br Med J 1928;1:12–3.

27. Klaiman MD, Shrader JA, Danoff JV, et al. Phonophoresis versus ultrasound in the treatment of common musculoskeletal conditions. Med Sci Sports Exerc 1998;30:1349–55.

28. Nirschl RP, Rodin DM, Ochiai DH, et al. Iontophoretic administration of dexamethasone sodium phosphate for acute epicondylitis. A randomized, double-blinded, placebo-controlled study. Am J Sports Med 2003;31(2):189–95.
29. Burnham R, Gregg R, Healy P, et al. The effectiveness of topical diclofenac for lateral epicondylitis. Clin J Sport Med 1998;8:78–81.
30. Altay T, Gunal I, Ozturk H. Local injection treatment for lateral epicondylitis. Clin Orthop 2001;398:127–30.
31. Solveborn A, Buch F, Mjallmin H, et al. Cortisone injection with anesthetic additive for radial epicondylagia (tennis elbow). Clin Orthop 1995;316:99–105.
32. Newcomer KL, Laskowski ER, Idank DM, et al. Corticosteroid injection in early treatment of lateral epicondylitis. Clin J Sport Med 2001;11:214–22.
33. Crowther MA, Bannister GC, Huma H, et al. A prospective, randomised study to compare extracorporeal shock-wave therapy and injection of steroid for the treatment of tennis elbow. J Bone Joint Surg Br 2002;84:678–9.
34. Verhaar JA, Walenkamp GH, van Mameren H, et al. Local corticosteroid injection versus Cyriax-type physiotherapy for tennis elbow. J Bone Joint Surg 1996;78:128–32.
35. Keizer SB, Rutten HP, Pilot P, et al. Botulinum toxin injection versus surgical treatment for tennis elbow. A randomized pilot study. Clin Orthop Relat Res 2002;401:125–31.
36. Walther M, Kirschner S, Koenig A, et al. Biomechanical evaluation of braces used for the treatment of epicondylitis. J Shoulder Elbow Surg 2002;11:265–70.
37. Ko JY, Chen HS, Chen LM. Treatment of lateral epicondylitis of the elbow with shock waves. Clin Orthop 2001;387:60–7.
38. Hammer DS, Supp S, Ensslin S, et al. Extracorporeal shock wave therapy in patients with tennis elbow and painful heel. Arch Orthop Trauma Surg 2000;120:304–7.
39. Rompe JD, Hopf C, Kullmer K, et al. Analgesic effect of extracorporeal shock-wave therapy on chronic tennis elbow. J Bone Joint Surg Br 1996;78:233–7.
40. Haake M, Konig IR, Decker T, et al. Extracorporeal shock wave therapy in the treatment of lateral epicondylitis. A randomized multicenter trial. J Bone Joint Surg 2002;84:1982–91.
41. Haake M, Boddeker IR, Decker T, et al. Side-effects of extracorporeal shock wave therapy in the treatment of tennis elbow. Arch Orthop Trauma Surg 2002;122:222–8.
42. Dlabach JA, Baker CL. Lateral and medial epicondylitis in the overhead athlete. Op Tech Orthop 2001;11:46–54.
43. Placzek R, Drescher W, Deuretzbacher G, et al. Treatment of chronic radial epicondylitis with botulinum toxin A. A double-blind, placebo-controlled, randomized multicenter study. J Bone Joint Surg Am 2007;89:255–60.
44. Peerbooms JC, Sluimer J, Bruijn DJ, et al. Positive effect of an autologous platelet concentrate in lateral epicondylitis in a double-blind randomized controlled trial. Platelet-rich plasma versus corticosteroid injection with a 1-year follow-up. Am J Sports Med 2010;38:255–62.
45. Mishra A, Pavelko T. Treatment of chronic elbow tendinosis with buffered platelet-rich plasma. Am J Sports Med 2006;34:1774–8.
46. Connell DA, Ali KE, Ahmad M, et al. Ultrasound-guided autologous blood injection for tennis elbow. Skeletal Radiol 2006;35:371–7.
47. Ul Gani N, Butt M, Dhar SA, et al. Autologous blood injection in the treatment of refractory tennis elbow. Internet J Orthop Surg 2007;5:1.

48. Rabago D, Best TM, Zgierska AE, et al. A systematic review of four injection therapies for lateral epicondylosis: prolotherapy, polidocanol, whole blood and platelet-rich plasma. Br J Sports Med 2009;43:471–81.
49. Scarpone M, Rabago DP, Zgierska A, et al. The efficacy of prolotherapy for lateral epicondylosis. Clin J Sport Med 2008;18:248–54.
50. Murrell GA. Using nitric oxide to treat tendinopathy. Br J Sports Med 2007;41: 227–31.
51. Paoloni JA, Appleyard RC, Nelson J, et al. Topical nitric oxide application in the treatment of chronic extensor tendinosis at the elbow: a randomized, double-blinded, placebo-controlled clinical trial. Am J Sports Med 2003;31:915–20.
52. Nirschl RP, Pettrone FA. Tennis elbow. The surgical treatment of lateral epicondylitis. J Bone Joint Surg Am 1979;61:832–9.
53. Boyd HB, McLeod AC. Tennis elbow. J Bone Joint Surg Am 1973;55:1183–7.
54. Baumgard SH, Schwartz DR. Percutaneous release of the epicondylar muscles for the humeral epicondylitis. Am J Sports Med 1982;10:233–6.
55. Dunkow PD, Jatti M, Muddu BN. A comparison of open and percutaneous techniques in the surgical treatment of tennis elbow. J Bone Joint Surg Br 2004;86: 701–4.
56. Grundberg AB, Dobson JF. Percutaneous release of the common extensor origin for tennis elbow. Clin Orthop Relat Res 2000;376:137–40.
57. Savoie FH III. Management of lateral epicondylitis with percutaneous release. Tech Shoulder Elbow Surg 2001;2:243–6.
58. Szabo SJ, Savoie FH 3rd, Field LD, et al. Tendinosis of the extensor carpi radialis brevis: an evaluation of three methods of operative treatment. J Shoulder Elbow Surg 2006;15:721–7.
59. Yerger B, Turner T. Percutaneous extensor tenotomy for chronic tennis elbow: an office procedure. Orthopedics 1985;8:1261–3.
60. Grifka J, Boenke S, Kramer J. Endoscopic therapy in epicondylitis radialis humeri. Arthroscopy 1995;11:743–8.
61. Rubenthaler F, Wiese M, Senge A, et al. Long term follow-up of open and endoscopic Hohmann procedures for lateral epicondylitis. Arthroscopy 2005;21: 684–90.
62. Goldberg EJ, Abraham E, Siegel I. The surgical treatment of chronic lateral humeral epicondylitis by common extensor release. Clin Orthop 1988;233: 208–12.
63. Hohmann G. Ober den Tennisellbogen. Verhandlungen der Deutschen Orthopädischen Gesellschaft 1927;21:349–54.
64. Verhaar J, Walenkamp G, Kester A, et al. Lateral extensor release for tennis elbow. J Bone Joint Surg Am 1993;75:1034–43.
65. Bosworth DM. The role of the orbicular ligament in tennis elbow. J Bone Joint Surg Am 1955;37:527–33.
66. Posch JN, Goldberg VM, Larrey R. Extensor fasciotomy for tennis elbow: a long term follow-up study. Clin Orthop Relat Res 1978;135:179–82.
67. Rayan GM, Coray SA. V-Y slide of the common extensor origin for lateral elbow tendinopathy. J Hand Surg Am 2001;26:1138–45.
68. Kaplan EB. Treatment of tennis elbow (epicondylitis) by denervation. J Bone Joint Surg Am 1959;41:147–51.
69. Wilhelm A. Tennis elbow: treatment of resistant cases by denervation. J Hand Surg Br 1996;21:523–33.
70. Almquist EE, Necking L, Bach AW. Epicondylar resection with aconeus muscle transfer for chronic lateral epicondylitis. J Hand Surg Am 1998;23:723–31.

71. Carroll RE, Jorgensen EC. Evaluation of the garden procedure for lateral epicondylitis. Clin Orthop Relat Res 1968;60:201–4.
72. Garden RS. Tennis elbow. J Bone Joint Surg Br 1961;43:100–6.
73. Stovell PB, Beinfield MS. Treatment of resistant lateral epicondylitis of the elbow by lengthening of the extensor carpi radialis brevis tendon. Surg Gynecol Obstet 1979;149:526–8.
74. Gardner RC. Tennis elbow: diagnosis, pathology and treatment. Nine severe cases treated by a new reconstructive operation. Clin Orthop Relat Res 1970; 72:248–53.
75. Khashaba A. Nirschl tennis elbow release with or without drilling. Br J Sports Med 2001;35:200–1.
76. Peart RE, Strickler SS, Schweitzer KM Jr. Lateral epicondylitis: a comparative study of open and arthroscopic lateral release. Am J Orthop 2004;33:565–7.
77. Zingg PO, Schneeberger AG. Debridement of extensors and drilling of the lateral epicondyle for tennis elbow: a retrospective study. J Shoulder Elbow Surg 2006;15:347–50.
78. Dunn JH, Kim JJ, Davis L, et al. Ten-to 14-year follow-up of the Nirschl surgical technique for lateral epicondylitis. Am J Sports Med 2008;36:261–6.
79. Thornton SJ, Rogers JR, Prickett WD, et al. Treatment of recalcitrant lateral epicondylitis with suture anchor repair. Am J Sports Med 2005;33:1558–64.
80. Rosenberg N, Henerdon I. Surgical treatment of resistant lateral epicondylitis: follow-up study of 19 patients after excision, release and repair of proximal common extensor tendon origin. Arch Orthop Trauma Surg 2002;122:514–7.
81. Baker CL, Murphy KP, Gottlob CA, et al. Arthroscopic classification and treatment of lateral epicondylitis: two-year clinical results. J Shoulder Elbow Surg 2000;9:475–82.
82. Baker CL Jr, Baker CL 3rd. Long-term follow-up of arthroscopic treatment of lateral epicondylitis. Am J Sports Med 2008;36:254–60.
83. Cummins CA. Lateral epicondylitis: in vivo assessment of arthroscopic debridement and correlation with patient outcomes. Am J Sports Med 2006;34: 1486–91.
84. Jerosch J, Schunck J. Arthroscopic treatment of lateral epicondylitis: indications, technique and early results. Knee Surg Sports Traumatol Arthrosc 2006; 14:379–82.
85. Mullett H, Sprague M, Brown G, et al. Arthroscopic treatment of lateral epicondylitis: clinical and cadaveric studies. Clin Orthop Relat Res 2005;439:123–8.
86. Owens BD, Murphy KP, Kuklo TR. Arthroscopic release for lateral epicondylitis. Arthroscopy 2001;17:582–7.
87. Romeo AA, Fox JA. Arthroscopic treatment of lateral epicondylitis: the 4-step technique. Orthop Tech Review 2002;4.
88. Sennoune B, Costa V, Dumontier C. Arthroscopic treatment of tennis elbow: preliminary experience with 14 patients. Rev Chir Orthop Reparatrice Appar Mot 2005;91:158–64.
89. Grewal R, MacDermid JC, Shah P, et al. Functional outcome of arthroscopic extensor carpi radialis brevis tendon release in chronic lateral epicondylitis. J Hand Surg Am 2009;34:849–57.
90. Cohen MS, Romeo AA, Hennigan SP, et al. Lateral epicondylitis: anatomic relationships of the extensor tendon origins and implications for arthroscopic treatment. J Shoulder Elbow Surg 2008;17:954–60.
91. Smith AM, Castle JA, Ruch DS. Arthroscopic resection of the common extensor origin: anatomic considerations. J Shoulder Elbow Surg 2003;12:375–9.

92. Kuklo TR, Taylor KF, Murphy KP, et al. Arthroscopic release for lateral epicondylitis: a cadaveric model. Arthroscopy 1999;15:259–64.
93. Ciccotti MC, Schwartz MA, Ciccotti MG. Diagnosis and treatment of medial epicondylitis of the elbow. Clin Sports Med 2004;23:693–705.
94. Glousman RE, Barron J, Jobe FW, et al. An electromyographic analysis of the elbow in normal and injured pitchers with medial collateral ligament insufficiency. Am J Sports Med 1992;20:311–7.
95. Chen FS, Rokito AS, Jobe FW. Medial elbow problems in the overhead-throwing athlete. J Am Acad Orthop Surg 2001;9:99–113.
96. Conway JE, Jobe FW, Glousman RE, et al. Medial instability of the elbow in throwing athletes. Treatment by repair or reconstruction of the ulnar collateral ligament. J Bone Joint Surg Am 1992;74:67–83.
97. Cain EL Jr, Dugas JR, Wolf RS, et al. Elbow injuries in throwing athletes: a current concepts review. Am J Sports Med 2003;31:621–35.
98. Callaway GH, Field LD, Deng XH, et al. Biomechanical evaluation of the medial collateral ligament of the elbow. J Bone Joint Surg Am 1997;79:1223–31.
99. Ollivierre CO, Nirschl RP, Pettrone FA. Resection and repair for medial tennis elbow. A prospective analysis. Am J Sports Med 1995;23:214–21.
100. Gabel GT, Morrey BF. Operative treatment of medical epicondylitis. Influence of concomitant ulnar neuropathy at the elbow. J Bone Joint Surg Am 1995;77:1065–9.
101. Richard MJ, Aldridge JM 3rd, Wiesler ER, et al. Traumatic valgus instability of the elbow: pathoanatomy and results of direct repair. J Bone Joint Surg Am 2008;90:2416–22.
102. Richard MJ, Aldridge JM 3rd, Wiesler ER, et al. Traumatic valgus instability of the elbow: pathoanatomy and results of direct repair. Surgical technique. J Bone Joint Surg Am 2009;91(Suppl 2):191–9.
103. Stahl S, Kaufman T. The efficacy of an injection of steroids for medial epicondylitis. A prospective study of sixty elbows. J Bone Joint Surg Am 1997;79:1648–52.
104. Stahl S, Kaufman T. Ulnar nerve injury at the elbow after steroid injection for medial epicondylitis. J Hand Surg Br 1997;22:69–70.
105. Kurvers H, Verhaar J. The results of operative treatment of medial epicondylitis. J Bone Joint Surg Am 1995;77:1374–9.
106. Vangsness CT Jr, Jobe FW. Surgical treatment of medial epicondylitis. Results in 35 elbows. J Bone Joint Surg Br 1991;73:409–11.

Acute Elbow Dislocations in Athletes

Bradford O. Parsons, MD[a],*, Matthew L. Ramsey, MD[b]

KEYWORDS

• Athlete • Elbow dislocation • Nonoperative treatment
• Surgical indications

DEFINITION

The elbow is the second most commonly dislocated joint in the body behind the shoulder in the adult population. In the pediatric patient population, the elbow is the most commonly dislocated joint. Simple dislocations represent dissociation of the ulnohumeral joint without concomitant fracture. Complex instability occurs when a fracture is associated with dislocation. Bony injuries associated with dislocation include radial head and neck fractures, coronoid fractures, and avulsion of the medial and/or lateral epicondyles. Additional injuries, remote from the elbow, occur in the forearm, wrist and hand, and shoulder.

Dislocations of the elbow in the athletic population are not uncommon. However, there is surprisingly little information about the management of these injuries in the athletic population. In particular, no specific guidelines for a return to play have been established. The treatment of simple dislocation of the elbow in athletes has been extrapolated from the treatments established for the general population.[1,2]

ANATOMY

Stability of the elbow is conferred by both the osseous and ligamentous anatomy of the joint. The primary osseous stabilizer of the elbow is the ulnohumeral joint composed of the trochlea, the coronoid and olecranon processes, and the greater sigmoid notch of the ulna. The primary ligamentous stabilizers of the elbow are the anterior band of the ulnar collateral ligament (aUCL) and the lateral ulnar collateral ligament (LUCL).[3,4] The origin of the aUCL is on the anterior inferior aspect of the medial epicondyle and it inserts on the sublime tubercle of the ulna (**Fig. 1**). The LUCL

[a] Department of Orthopaedic Surgery, Mount Sinai School of Medicine, One Gustave L. Levy Place, PO Box 1188, New York, NY 10029, USA
[b] Shoulder and Elbow Service, Rothman Institute, Department of Orthopaedic Surgery, Thomas Jefferson University, 925 Chestnut Street, Philadelphia, PA 19107, USA
* Corresponding author.
E-mail address: Bradford.parsons@mountsinai.org

Clin Sports Med 29 (2010) 599–609
doi:10.1016/j.csm.2010.06.005
0278-5919/10/$ – see front matter © 2010 Elsevier Inc. All rights reserved.

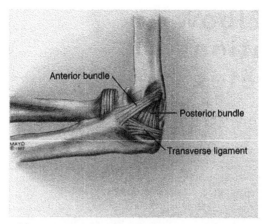

Fig. 1. The anatomy of the UCL. The anterior bundle of the aUCL is the primary valgus stabilizer of the elbow. (*Reprinted from* Morrey BF. Anatomy of the elbow joint. In: Morrey BF, Sanchez-Sotelo J, editors. The elbow and its disorders. 4th edition. Philadelphia: Saunders Elsevier; 2009. p. 21; with permission.)

originates from an isometric point on the lateral epicondyle and travels across the inferior aspect of the radial head before inserting on the supinator crest of the ulna (**Fig. 2**).[5] The radial head is a secondary static stabilizer, and the flexor-pronator and common extensor muscles of the forearm are secondary dynamic stabilizers of the elbow.

PATHOANATOMY

O'Driscoll and colleagues[3] coined the term posterolateral rotatory instability (PLRI) to describe the sequence of pathologic events culminating in ulnohumeral dislocation.

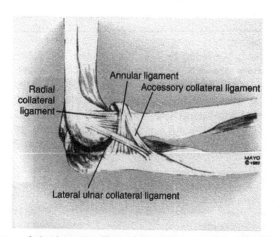

Fig. 2. The anatomy of the lateral collateral ligament complex. The LUCL portion of the lateral collateral ligament complex is the primary lateral soft tissue restraint to posterolateral rotatory instability (PLRI). (*Reprinted from* Morrey BF. Anatomy of the elbow joint. In: Morrey BF, Sanchez-Sotelo J, editors. The elbow and its disorders. 4th edition. Philadelphia: Saunders Elsevier; 2009. p. 22; with permission.)

PLRI is caused by a fall on an outstretched arm resulting in progressive capsular injury (**Fig. 3**). As the body rotates around a fixed hand, external rotation and valgus moments are generated, which initially disrupts the LUCL (Stage I). As the capsular injury progresses medially with tearing of the anterior and posterior capsules, the ulna can perch on the distal humerus (Stage II). Dislocation occurs in 2 stages. In the first stage of dislocation (Stage IIIA) all of the soft tissues are torn up to, but not including, the aUCL. In stage IIIB, the ulnar collateral ligament (UCL) is disrupted (**Fig. 4**).[6]

Simple elbow dislocations are classified by the direction of displacement as posterior, anterior, or divergent based on the relationship of the ulna and radius to the humerus. The most common direction of dislocation is posterior with the forearm positioned either medial or lateral to the humerus. Anterior and divergent dislocations are rare in comparison to posterior dislocations.

HISTORY AND PHYSICAL EXAMINATION

The history following an acute elbow dislocation is directed toward determining the timeline and mechanism of injury, presence of recurrent episodes of instability, frequency of dislocations, and previous treatment.

Physical examination at the time of evaluation requires a careful neurovascular assessment. Nerve injury can occur following elbow dislocation, and a thorough neurologic examination of the extremity is mandatory prior to any treatment of the dislocation. The ulnar nerve is most frequently involved, although median or radial nerve injury may also occur.[7]

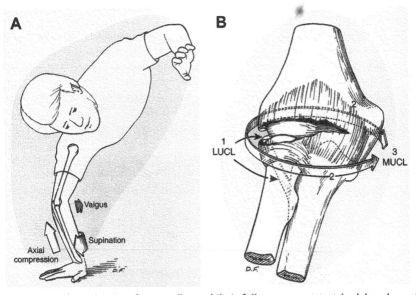

Fig. 3. Proposed mechanism for an elbow. (*A*) A fall on an outstretched hand creates angular and rotational forces, resulting in failure of the LUCL. (*B*) Soft tissue disruption progresses toward the medial elbow with failure of the anterior and posterior capsule. Disruption of the UCL results in elbow dislocation. (*Reprinted from* O'Driscoll SW. Elbow dislocations. In: Morrey BF, Sanchez-Sotelo J, editors. The elbow and its disorders. 4th edition. Philadelphia: Saunders Elsevier; 2009. p. 437, 438; with permission.)

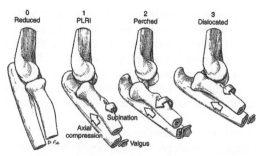

Fig. 4. Clinical stages of elbow instability that correlate with the stages of soft tissue disruption. (*Reprinted from* O'Driscoll SW. Elbow dislocations. In: Morrey BF, Sanchez-Sotelo J, editors. The elbow and its disorders. 4th edition. Philadelphia: Saunders Elsevier; 2009. p. 437, 438; with permission.)

Examination of the dislocated elbow demonstrates obvious deformity, with the elbow often held in a varus position and the forearm supinated.

Physical examination must include an assessment of the shoulder, forearm, and wrist for associated injuries.

IMAGING AND OTHER DIAGNOSTIC STUDIES

Standard orthogonal radiographs of the elbow usually provide sufficient information to evaluate the injury pattern and assess for associated fracture (**Fig. 5**). If a radial head fracture is identified in association with an elbow dislocation, a coronoid fracture should be assumed until proved otherwise. Postreduction radiographs confirm relocation of the joint (**Fig. 6**). The congruency of the ulnohumeral and radiocapitellar joints is carefully assessed. Stress radiographs are rarely of value in determining treatment.

Computed tomography scans with 3-dimensional reconstructions are obtained in any situation where a fracture may be suspected, because it is critical to identify fractures, which may be an indication for surgical management. Magnetic resonance imaging has very little role in acute elbow dislocations.

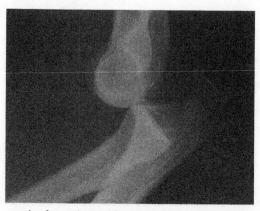

Fig. 5. Lateral radiograph of a patient with posterolateral dislocation of the elbow.

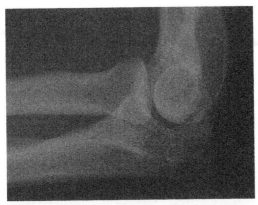

Fig. 6. Lateral radiograph following reduction of a posterolateral dislocation of the elbow. Note the concentric reduction of the ulnohumeral and radiocapitellar joints.

ACUTE MANAGEMENT OF ELBOW DISLOCATION

Reduction of the elbow often requires some form of anesthesia. Conscious sedation is usually adequate to obtain enough relaxation to atraumatically reduce the elbow. The patient is placed supine with the arm overhead. The dislocation is reduced by recreating the deformity that resulted in the dislocation. For posterior dislocations occurring as a result of the posterolateral rotatory mechanism, the elbow is hypersupinated to clear the coronoid from the distal humerus and then extended with a valgus stress applied. Pushing the olecranon distally then reduces the joint. Reduction is often noticed by a palpable clunk. Once reduction is achieved, the elbow is flexed and the forearm pronated. The forearm is maintained in pronation to hinge the elbow closed on the UCL if intact. If reduction cannot be achieved or maintained, open reduction and soft tissue repair or reconstruction is required.

After initial reduction, the neurovascular status of the limb is reevaluated. Although the loss of neurologic function after closed reduction is rare, its presence can be an indication for surgical exploration to rule out nerve entrapment. Stability of the joint is assessed based on the amount of extension obtainable before instability is encountered and the association of pronation with instability. Assessment of postreduction stability can be difficult in the awake patient. It is helpful to assess stability throughout the range of motion (ROM) while the patient is still sedated or anesthetized.

With the forearm pronated, the elbow is assessed for varus, valgus, and rotatory instability. If the elbow is stable throughout the arc of motion, it is immobilized in a sling or splint. If instability is present as the elbow is brought into extension, the forearm is pronated to hinge the elbow closed on the UCL. If the elbow subluxes in less than 30° flexion with the forearm pronated, it is splinted in 90° of flexion and neutral rotation. If the elbow remains concentrically reduced, the arm is maintained splinted. If instability persists, surgery to repair the soft issue constraint may be an option to confer stability to the elbow. Assessment of the lateral radiograph for a "drop sign" is critical, as it carries a high risk of recurrent instability (**Fig. 7**).[8]

NONOPERATIVE MANAGEMENT

Once a stable reduction is obtained, most simple dislocations can be managed nonoperatively with splinting or bracing, guided by the degree of instability determined during postreduction examination. If the elbow is stable throughout an arc of motion,

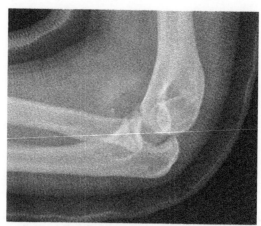

Fig. 7. Postreduction lateral radiograph demonstrating a "drop" sign. The widening of the ulnohumeral joint and the position of the radial head on the inferior aspect of the capitalism should be noted. (*Reprinted from* Duckworth A, Ring D, Kulijdian A, et al. Unstable elbow dislocations. J Shoulder Elbow Surg 2008;17(2):283; with permission.)

it is immobilized in a sling or splint for 3 to 5 days for comfort and then ROM exercises are begun. If instability is present moving into extension but remains stable into flexion, the elbow is braced with an extension block about 10° above the point in extension where instability is encountered. Careful review of postreduction radiographs should demonstrate a concentrically reduced joint. Occasionally, there is slight widening of the joint noted on postreduction radiographs without frank dislocation. In a select group of carefully followed patients, muscle activation exercises have been shown to dynamically stabilize the joint.[9] Weekly radiographs are needed to ensure maintenance of a congruent joint during the first few weeks following injury. If bracing is used, it can typically be discontinued 3 to 4 weeks following injury and terminal stretching begun to regain motion.

SURGICAL MANAGEMENT
Indications

Surgical management of simple elbow dislocation is indicated in elbows that remain unstable, even when placed in flexion and pronation. These elbows typically have extensive soft tissue injury involving the lateral and UCLs, the common extensor and flexor-pronator muscle attachments, and the anterior capsule. Surgical stabilization of the elbow typically requires ligament repair. However, ligament reconstruction is occasionally required.

Disruption of the LUCL is the critical lesion of dislocation, and therefore is addressed first. The LUCL usually avulses from its origin at the lateral epicondyle, often leaving a "bald" epicondyle (**Fig. 8**). Repair of the LUCL to the epicondyle is usually sufficient and may be performed via bone tunnels in the humerus or with suture anchors, depending on surgeon preference. Reconstruction of the LUCL is rarely needed in the acute setting but is required in cases of chronic instability.

Repair or reconstruction of the LUCL frequently reestablishes stability, even in the face of disruption of the UCL, because the intact radial head, acting as a secondary stabilizer, resists valgus instability. Persistent instability despite repair or reconstruction of the LUCL requires stabilization of the UCL.

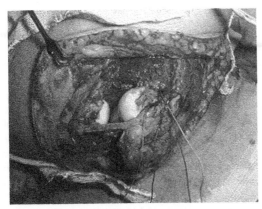

Fig. 8. Intraoperative photograph in a patient with an unstable elbow dislocation. Note the absence of soft tissue attachments to the lateral epicondyle that indicates a "bald" epicondyle. (*Reprinted from* Duckworth A, Ring D, Kulijdian A, et al. Unstable elbow dislocations. J Shoulder Elbow Surg 2008;17(2):282; with permission.)

Following collateral ligament repair or reconstruction, the common extensor and flexor-pronator masses are repaired to their epicondylar attachments. In the rare circumstance when the elbow remains unstable despite surgical management of the LUCL, UCL, and tendon origins, a static or hinged external fixator is required to maintain the reduced joint.

SURGICAL TECHNIQUE
Patient Positioning

Patients are positioned supine with the arm extended on a radiolucent hand table. A small bump is placed under the ipsilateral scapula. The arm is draped free to permit the entire brachium to remain in the surgical field. A sterile tourniquet is applied to the brachium. If the use of autograft is anticipated for ligament reconstruction, the hand and/or leg are prepped for harvest of palmaris longus or hamstring tendon, respectively.

Surgical Approach and Arthrotomy

Two different superficial approaches can be used to gain exposure to the deep fascial intervals of the lateral and medial elbow. A posterior midline skin incision with medial and lateral subcutaneous flaps provides access to the deeper intervals and allows extensile exposure if needed. Alternatively, separate lateral and medial incisions can be used. There are benefits to both approaches, and currently no data exist establishing the superiority of one approach over the other.

The authors prefer a separate lateral and, if necessary, a medial incision. The lateral elbow is approached through Kocher interval between the anconeus and extensor carpi ulnaris (ECU). The fascia at Kocher interval is split, exposing the degree of soft tissue injury at the lateral epicondyle. In patients with persistent instability following simple dislocation, the lateral soft tissues are often avulsed from their bony origin, presenting a bald epicondyle (see **Fig. 8**). The anconeus and ECU are elevated from the lateral capsule and the torn LUCL is identified. The posterior interosseous nerve (PIN) is at risk with this exposure, and therefore the forearm is kept pronated to protect the PIN. The radial head and coronoid are inspected to confirm no fractures are present. Similarly, the distal humeral articular surface is evaluated for occult chondral injury.

Ligament Repair

The origin of the LUCL is identified at the lateral epicondyle. In most cases, a sleeve of tissue is avulsed from the lateral epicondyle including the LUCL. The location of the ligament at the radiocapitellar joint can be identified by a fold of tissue on the deep surface of the capsule that identifies the location of the joint. A suture anchor or divergent drill holes at the lateral epicondyle are used to secure the ligament to the epicondyle. Drill holes are preferred as they facilitate a more stable repair of both the collateral ligament and the common extensor mass. A running number 2 nonabsorbable Krakow locking stitch is placed along the anterior and posterior aspect of the LUCL starting at the origin of the ligament. The suture/ligament construct is tensioned to confirm integrity of the insertion of the LUCL onto the ulna. Drill holes are made at the ligament attachment and the sutures are passed through bone (**Fig. 9**).

The joint is reduced and the sutures are tensioned with the arm in 30° of flexion and neutral rotation. The suture is clamped but not tied until a concentric reduction is confirmed fluoroscopically. The elbow is taken through an arc of motion to assess stability. If the elbow is stable through an arc of motion, the suture is tied and the common extensor origin is repaired using the suture used to repair the ligament. If the elbow remains unstable, particularly moving toward full extension, the UCL must be addressed. In this situation, the lateral soft tissue repair is not tied until the medial repair is completed.

A medial skin incision centered on the medial epicondyle is used. Subcutaneous flaps are elevated with the cutaneous nerves identified and protected. The deep approach to the aUCL depends on the extent of injury to the flexor-pronator mass. There is often a significant injury to the flexor-pronator mass. In this case, the aUCL can be approached through the flexor-pronator defect. Similar to the lateral side, the aUCL can be repaired using bone tunnels or a suture anchor placed at the origin of the ligament at the anterior inferior aspect of the medial epicondyle. A Krakow suture is placed in the aUCL and passed through drill holes in the medial epicondyle (**Fig. 10**).

Once all of the sutures are placed, they are tied beginning on the lateral side of the elbow with the joint concentrically reduced. The elbow is placed in 30° of flexion and the forearm in neutral rotation. Care must be taken not to overtighten the lateral side, as this results in medial joint gapping. Once the LUCL repair is completed, the aUCL repair is completed with the elbow in 30° of flexion and neutral forearm rotation. The common extensor and flexor-pronator masses are repaired to the lateral and medial

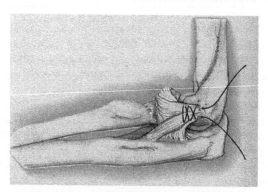

Fig. 9. Repair of the LUCL and lateral collateral ligament complex through drill holes in the lateral epicondyle. (*Reprinted from* Morrey BF. Chronic unreduced elbow dislocation. In: Morrey BF, Sanchez-Sotelo J, editors. The elbow and its disorders. 4th edition. Philadelphia: Saunders Elsevier; 2009. p. 466; with permission.)

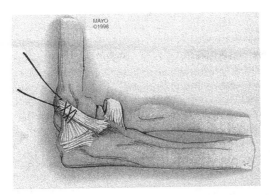

Fig. 10. Repair of the anterior bundle of the aUCL through drill holes in the anterior inferior aspect of the medial epicondyle. (*Reprinted from* Morrey BF. Chronic unreduced elbow dislocation. In: Morrey BF, Sanchez-Sotelo J, editors. The elbow and its disorders. 4th edition. Philadelphia: Saunders Elsevier; 2009. p. 466; with permission.)

epicondyle, respectively. The fascia of Kocher interval is securely closed, which provides additional rotational stability to the elbow. Wound closure is performed in standard fashion.

If the elbow remains unstable after repair of the LUCL and aUCL, a hinged or static external fixator must be applied (**Fig. 11**).

POSTOPERATIVE CARE

Following surgery the elbow is splinted in flexion for 3 to 5 days to allow for wound healing. ROM exercises are then begun in flexion, extension, and rotation, with care taken to avoid varus or valgus stress. Although not mandatory, a hinged orthosis can be helpful in protecting the ligament repair/reconstruction. Active assisted and gentle passive motion is continued for 6 weeks. Strengthening is begun 4 to 6 weeks following surgery.

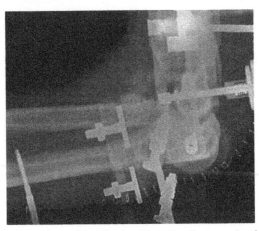

Fig. 11. Radiograph of a patient with a simple dislocation that remained unstable following lateral and medial soft tissue repair. Not the application of a hinged external fixator to maintain the elbow concentrically reduced. (*Reprinted from* Duckworth AD, Ring D, Kulijdian A, et al. Unstable elbow dislocations. J Shoulder Elbow Surg 2008;17(2):283; with permission.)

OUTCOMES

The management of simple dislocations of the elbow is well established in the literature and is primarily based on the stability of the elbow following reduction. Several studies have established nonoperative management of the elbow with a short period of immobilization. Josefsson and colleagues[10,11] performed 2 studies evaluating the results of surgical and nonsurgical management of simple dislocations. The nature of the soft tissue injuries was identified at the time of surgery and included injury to the UCL, with or without injury to the lateral collateral ligament and variable injury to the flexor-pronator and common extensor tendons. Josefsson and colleagues found no difference between the patients treated with surgical repair of the disrupted soft tissues or those treated nonoperatively. The most common problem following either treatment was loss of extension.

The length of immobilization following reduction has been directly related to the final outcome. Mehlhoff and colleagues[12] demonstrated that immobilization for longer than 3 weeks was associated with persistent loss of extension. Similarly, Eygendaal and colleagues[13] reported the long-term results in patients following closed management of simple dislocations. The majority of patients (62%) described their elbow function as good or excellent. However, many patients experienced mild loss of extension. The literature clearly supports a shorter period of immobilization to prevent disability.

The surgical management of recurrent instability has been reported in several series. While many of the patients in these studies had fractures associated with dislocation (complex instability), many had isolated soft tissue injuries. The results of a group of patients with postreduction instability treated with ligament and tendon repair were reported by Micic and colleagues.[14] Injury to the medial and lateral ligamentous and tendon structures were encountered and surgically managed. The patients had mild loss of terminal extension with overall good results. No patient required further surgery. Nestor and colleagues[15] reported a select group of patients with recurrent PLRI managed with either repair or reconstruction of the LUCL. An excellent result was obtained in 7 of 11 (64%) patients and 10 of 11 (91%) remained stable. Other investigators have found more predictable results with ligament reconstruction compared with ligament repair in patients with chronic PLRI.[16] More recently, Sanchez-Sotelo and colleagues[17] reported the results of 44 patients treated for recurrent PLRI. Instability occurred after simple dislocation in 9 patients. Overall, 32 (75%) of patients had an excellent result based on the Mayo Elbow Performance Score.

Most patients with a simple dislocation are successfully managed with a short period of immobilization followed by early ROM. The unique challenge in the athletic population is determining return to sports participation without fear of recurrent injury. The literature does not specifically guide this decision. However, Protzman[18] provided insight into this issue. He reported the experience with elbow dislocation at the United States Military Academy. This patient population engages in strenuous activities in the course of their training and represents an athletic population. The results of treatment were evaluated with respect to the duration of immobilization. Regardless of the period of immobilization, all patients had normal flexion, pronation, and supination. The patients who were immobilized for less than 5 days had 3° loss of extension and 6 weeks of disability before returning to full active duty. Longer periods of immobilization lead to greater loss of extension and a longer period of disability.

SUMMARY

Simple dislocations of the elbow occur in the athletic population. Initial management of a simple dislocation in an athlete does not differ from that of the general population.

The major difference in the athletic population is the appropriate time to return to sports participation. Early return to activities is supported in the literature. A short period of immobilization followed by progressive ROM and strengthening is followed by early return to activities.

REFERENCES

1. Plancher KD, Lucas TS. Fracture dislocations of the elbow in athletes. Clin Sports Med 2001;20(1):59–76.
2. Rettig AC. Traumatic elbow injuries in the athlete. Orthop Clin North Am 2002; 33(3):509–22, v.
3. O'Driscoll SW, Bell DF, Morrey BF. Posterolateral rotatory instability of the elbow. J Bone Joint Surg 1991;73(3):440–6.
4. Morrey BF, Tanaka S, An KN. Valgus stability of the elbow. A definition of primary and secondary constraints. Clin Orthop Relat Res 1991;265:187–95.
5. Morrey BF, An KN. Functional anatomy of the ligaments of the elbow. Clin Orthop Relat Res 1985;201:84–90.
6. O'Driscoll SW, Morrey BF, Korinek S, et al. Elbow subluxation and dislocation. A spectrum of instability. Clin Orthop Relat Res 1992;280:186–97.
7. Rana NA, Kenwright J, Taylor RG, et al. Complete lesion of the median nerve associated with dislocation of the elbow joint. Acta Orthop Scand 1974;45(3): 365–9.
8. Coonrad RW, Roush TF, Major NM, et al. The drop sign, a radiographic warning sign of elbow instability. J Shoulder Elbow Surg 2005;14(3):312–7.
9. Duckworth AD, Kulijdian A, McKee MD, et al. Residual subluxation of the elbow after dislocation or fracture-dislocation: treatment with active elbow exercises and avoidance of varus stress. J Shoulder Elbow Surg 2008;17(2):276–80.
10. Josefsson PO, Gentz CF, Johnell O, et al. Surgical versus non-surgical treatment of ligamentous injuries following dislocation of the elbow joint. A prospective randomized study. J Bone Joint Surg 1987;69(4):605–8.
11. Josefsson PO, Gentz CF, Johnell O, et al. Surgical versus nonsurgical treatment of ligamentous injuries following dislocations of the elbow joint. Clin Orthop Relat Res 1987;214:165–9.
12. Mehlhoff TL, Noble PC, Bennett JB, et al. Simple dislocation of the elbow in the adult. Results after closed treatment. J Bone Joint Surg 1988;70(2):244–9.
13. Eygendaal D, Verdegaal SH, Obermann WR, et al. Posterolateral dislocation of the elbow joint. Relationship to medial instability. J Bone Joint Surg 2000;82(4): 555–60.
14. Micic I, Kim SY, Park IH, et al. Surgical management of unstable elbow dislocation without intra-articular fracture. Int Orthop 2009;33:1141–7.
15. Nestor BJ, O'Driscoll SW, Morrey BF. Ligamentous reconstruction for posterolateral rotatory instability of the elbow. J Bone Joint Surg 1992;74(8):1235–41.
16. Lee BP, Teo LH. Surgical reconstruction for posterolateral rotatory instability of the elbow. J Shoulder Elbow Surg 2003;12(5):476–9.
17. Sanchez-Sotelo J, Morrey BF, O'Driscoll SW. Ligamentous repair and reconstruction for posterolateral rotatory instability of the elbow. J Bone Joint Surg 2005;87(1):54–61.
18. Protzman RR. Dislocation of the elbow joint. J Bone Joint Surg 1978;60(4): 539–41.

Arthroscopic and Open Radial Ulnohumeral Ligament Reconstruction for Posterolateral Rotatory Instability of the Elbow

Felix H. Savoie III, MD[a,*], Michael J. O'Brien, MD[a],
Larry D. Field, MD[b], Daniel J. Gurley, MD[c]

KEYWORDS

- Elbow • Instability • Posterolateral instability of the elbow
- Arthroscopy

There has been a growing interest in the diagnosis and treatment of posterolateral rotatory instability (PLRI) of the elbow since the original description by O'Driscoll and colleagues in 1991.[1] PLRI has been described as an instability pattern of the elbow that results from an incompetent radial ulnohumeral ligament complex (RUHL) (**Fig. 1**).[1] Subsequent to the original description by O'Driscoll and colleagues,[1] numerous anatomic studies have attempted to further define the involved tissue. Dunning and colleagues[2] stated that both the RUHL and the radial collateral ligament (RCL) must be sectioned to achieve PLRI. They also stated that they could not differentiate visually the 2 ligaments at their humeral origin. They could only differentiate the RUHL from the RCL by identifying the distal extent of the RUHL at the supinator crest of the ulna. Seki and colleagues[3] were able to show that sectioning just the anterior band of the lateral collateral complex induced instability. This suggests that an intact RUHL cannot stabilize the elbow. These data demonstrate that the entity of PLRI is in fact a spectrum of injury. Although originally described as sequelae of an elbow

[a] Department of Orthopaedic Surgery, Tulane Institute of Sports Medicine, Tulane University, 1430 Tulane Avenue, SL-32, New Orleans, LA 70112, USA
[b] Upper Extremity Service, Mississippi Sports Medicine and Orthopaedic Center, 1325 East Fortification Street, Jackson, MS 39202, USA
[c] College Park Family Care Center, 10600 Mastin, Overland Park, KS 66212, USA
* Corresponding author.
E-mail address: Fsavoie@tulane.edu

Clin Sports Med 29 (2010) 611–618
doi:10.1016/j.csm.2010.06.008
0278-5919/10/$ – see front matter © 2010 Elsevier Inc. All rights reserved.

sportsmed.theclinics.com

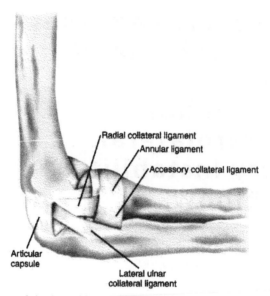

Radial collateral ligament
Annular ligament
Accessory collateral ligament
Articular capsule
Lateral ulnar collateral ligament

Fig. 1. The anatomy of the lateral ligamentous complex is demonstrated.

dislocation, these anatomic studies help support our own experience that there is a continuum of injury between PLRI and frank elbow dislocation.[1,4]

This instability is best demonstrated clinically with the pivot shift test of the elbow. This test, as first described by O'Driscoll and colleagues,[1] may elicit gross instability or simply pain and apprehension. Two other clinical tests, described by Regan and Lapner,[5] produce pain when pushing up from (1) an arm chair with the palms facing inward and (2) a prone position, first with the forearms maximally pronated and with the thumbs pointing toward each other, then with the thumbs pointed outward and the forearms maximally supinated, which causes symptoms that were not present with the forearms pronated. Alternately, this can be performed standing while performing a wall push-up.[5]

Imaging studies for PLRI may be helpful. In the acute situation, radiographs may reveal an avulsion fragment from the humeral lateral epicondyle. Often, however, radiographs are normal. A stress radiograph or fluoroscopy while performing the pivot shift test will show the radial head and proximal ulnar moving together to a subluxated, posterolaterally rotated position. This is best performed under anesthesia, however. Magnetic resonance imaging of the elbow has been described to identify a lesion in the RUHL.[6] MR arthrography may be more useful in defining the pathology associated with lateral-sided instability, but a negative test does not automatically rule out PLRI.[4] The last diagnostic modality may be direct arthroscopic visualization of the instability, with laxity of the annular ligament and the demonstration of the arthroscopic "drive-through sign" (**Fig. 2**).[7,8]

INDICATIONS FOR SURGERY

The indication for surgery for PLRI is the same as for any problem: pain and functional limitation. The key decision making in PLRI is recognition of the pathology and the determination of the best available technique to restore function. In most acute and subacute injuries, a repair, either arthroscopic or open techniques, will provide the optimal method of recovery. In the chronic or revision cases, one should plan to

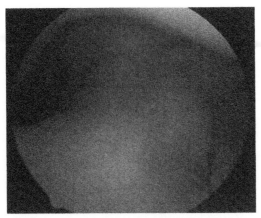

Fig. 2. The posterolateral "drive-through" sign of the lateral gutter present in posterolateral instability is demonstrated in this view.

add plication sutures in addition to anchoring the ligaments back to the epicondyle via anchors or drill holes. A graft should be considered in cases in which there is no palpable soft tissue over the radio-capitellar joint, multiply operated elbows, an absent anconeus muscle, and in cases in which the MR arthrogram shows no ligamentous tissue available to use for a repair.

We believe most primary cases are amenable to arthroscopic repair and plication no matter the duration of the dysfunction. This is our procedure of choice for both primary PLRI and in all cases in which a prior ligament reconstruction has not been attempted. We have found the arthroscopic technique to be especially beneficial in revision lateral epicondylitis surgery when there was most likely an instability component before the index lateral epicondylitis procedure. In patients with prior ligament revision surgery, the quality of tissue available often becomes more problematic, and we usually have consent for graft harvest or allograft tissue before beginning the procedure. A diagnostic arthroscopy to confirm the instability and a view of the postero-lateral gutter will confirm the paucity of tissue and allow easy conversion to an open reconstructive procedure.

SURGICAL TECHNIQUES
Open Repair

There are 2 open methods used in the management of PLRI: repair achieved with 1 or more suture anchors or reconstruction with a free tendon graft. Patients who are identified to have a bony avulsion from the lateral epicondyle can be managed by open repair of the avulsion fracture back to the humerus. The usual location for anchor placement is on the distal posterior aspect of the lateral epicondyle. The repaired ligament should be tightened with the elbow flexed to 60° to prevent overtightening of the repair with subsequent loss of flexion (**Fig. 3**A).

Patients with a palpable defect in their extensor mass tendon in addition to the tear can be treated with an open repair of both the ligament and the tendon.

Open Reconstruction with Graft

Patients in which there is insufficient tissue require a free tendon graft to correct the instability. This is best accomplished by placing the midportion of the graft into a tunnel

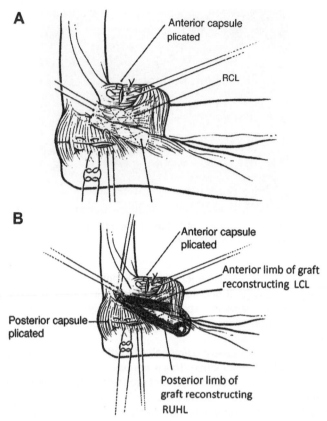

Fig. 3. (*A*) Open repair of the lateral ligaments with plication of the bands and repair of the complex back to the humerus can be accomplished in patients with lateral instability. (*B*) Reconstruction of the lateral ligaments via a graft technique using an interference screw in the ulna and docking to the humerus.

in the supinator crest of the ulna and fixating it with an interference screw. One limb of the graft is placed under the annular ligament and then up to the distal end of the lateral epicondyle to re-create the lateral collateral ligament (LCL) component and add to the stability of the annular ligament. The other limb is placed directly under the anconeus and docked into the posterior epicondyle in the isometric point described by O'Driscoll and colleagues[1] (see **Fig. 3**B).

Arthroscopic Repair

The development of an arthroscopic technique for the treatment of PLRI was described by Smith and colleagues[4] in 2001. The instability can be readily seen during arthroscopic evaluation. While viewing from the proximal anteromedial portal, the ulna and radial head can be seen to subluxate posterolaterally during the performance of a pivot shift test. Additionally, an arthroscope in the posterolateral portal can be driven through the lateral gutter and into the lateral aspect of the ulnohumeral joint. The ability to drive the arthroscope into the ulnohumeral joint is analogous to the "drive-through sign" in shoulder instability (see **Fig. 2**). Additionally, this view is not attainable in stable elbows or after the instability is corrected in patients with PLRI.

The instability from a lax LCL complex can be effectively treated with an arthroscopic plication. This is performed by placing 4 to 7 absorbable sutures into the postero-lateral gutter from the radial border of the ulna via a spinal needle from distal to proximal. Each suture is then retrieved proximally out along the humerus using a retrograde retriever. The first suture is delivered into the joint through the annular ligament (**Fig. 4**A). Subsequent sutures are brought into the joint in a progressively more proximal position. Each suture is immediately retrieved with a suture retriever that passes into the joint adjacent to the lateral epicondyle (see **Fig. 4**B). These sutures are then retrieved subcutaneously through one skin portal and pulled to tension. The arthroscope is driven out of the lateral gutter as the sutures are tensioned. The sutures are then tied individually from distal to proximal. If there is laxity or subluxation still present after the sutures are pretensioned, an anchor can be placed at the isometric point of the lateral epicondyle and 1 limb of suture can pass under all of the loops of the plication sutures to a retriever over the suture to afford greater overall tension on the plication and repair the reconstructed complex to the humerus (see **Fig. 4**C).

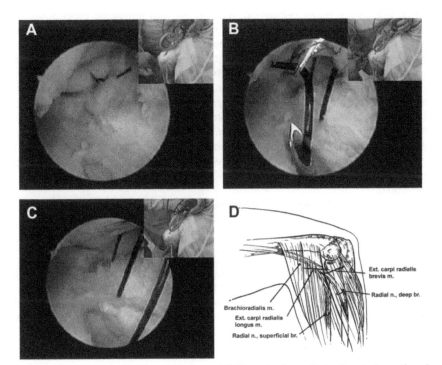

Fig. 4. The arthroscopic plication technique: (*A*) The spinal needle is placed along the ulna into the posterolateral gutter under the annular ligament, and a passing suture is placed through it into the joint, beginning the plication. (*B*) A retrograde retriever is placed along the posterior aspect of the lateral epicondyle and used to retrieve the suture, leaving the suture aligned from distal posterior to anterior superior, to tighten and plicate the RUHL complex. (*C*) Steps "A" and "B" are repeated, moving proximally until multiple sutures are in place plicating the RUHL. The entire complex is then repaired to the humerus using an anchor and suture combination. (*D*) The radial nerve (*yellow*), the surrounding musculature, and the approximate location of the safe access sites (*red*) for the placement of the retrograde retriever and spinal needle during arthroscopic reconstruction are illustrated.

In all cases, one should be cognizant of the location of the radial nerve and its branches as well as the lateral ante-brachial cutaneous nerve. Suture retrieval is always done posterior to the most anterior aspect of the lateral epicondyle and always proximal to the radial head to avoid inadvertent damage to the nerve (see **Fig. 4**D).

Postoperatively, patients are immediately immobilized in a fiberglass splint with the forearm rotation at neutral and the elbow at 0° to 30° of extension. This is progressed in the first week to a double-hinged elbow brace with the arc of motion from 0° to 45° for approximately 2 more weeks. The motion is slowly increased in 10° to 20° increments over the next 5 weeks until a functional arc of motion is achieved. Six weeks postoperatively, most patients will begin wrist and elbow strengthening exercises in the brace. Approximately 8 weeks after surgery, the brace can be removed for activities of daily living. Depending on individual progression, patients are allowed to start strengthening exercises out of brace at 10 to 12 weeks. They must be able to perform all strengthening exercises pain-free in the brace before progression out of the brace.

RESULTS

In a previous report, Savoie and colleagues[8] reported on 61 patients (**Table 1**). All patients had a PLRI repair performed, and several had additional procedures performed. Sixteen had a concurrent lateral epicondylitis procedure, 6 had an open extensor mass avulsion repair, and 4 were treated with an open posterior interosseous nerve release. Three of the patients treated by open means had a reconstruction performed with a free tendon graft. The other 34 open procedures had a suture repair of the lateral collateral ligamentous complex. Six of the 17 arthroscopically treated patients had the addition of an anchor to supplement the arthroscopic suture plication.

The average follow-up was 41 months (range 12–103 months). Overall Andrews-Carson scores for all repairs improved from 145 to 180 ($P<.0001$).[9] Subjective scores improved from 57 to 85 ($P<.0001$) and objective scores improved from 88 to 95 ($P = .008$). Subdividing the technique yielded these overall results: arthroscopic repairs improved from 146 to 176 ($P = .0001$) and open repairs from 144 to 182 ($P<.001$).

In O'Driscoll and colleagues'[1] initial report of 5 cases, 2 patients were managed by repair and 3 by grafting.

DISCUSSION

The diagnosis of posterolateral instability has become more common since the original description by O'Driscoll and colleagues.[1] Numerous studies have helped delineate the mechanism of injury that produces the various kinds of lateral instability. Reports by Regan and Lapner[5] and others[7,8,10] have addressed the examination

Table 1							
Results from Savoie and colleagues[8]							
	Subjective		Objective		Overall		
Andrews-Carson Scores	**Preop**	**Postop**	**Preop**	**Postop**	**Preop**	**Postop**	**Average Follow-up, mo**
Arthroscopic	55	83	91	93	146	176	33
Open	58	86	86	96	144	182	44
Total	57	85	88	95	145	180	41

Abbreviations: Postop, postoperative; Preop, preoperative.

techniques useful in making the clinical diagnosis. Our own studies have shown the success that can be achieved in most cases with arthroscopic repair and plication of the RUHL.

It was interesting to note that in the Savoie and colleagues'[8] series, 25% of patients had a previous lateral epicondylar repair surgery. Kalainov and Cohen[10] reported on the coexistence of PLRI and lateral epicondylitis. Although PLRI is an uncommon diagnosis and the repair procedure is not commonly performed, tennis elbow releases are executed by most orthopedic surgeons. Treating surgeons should be aware of the differential diagnosis of lateral elbow pain. This includes PLRI, lateral epicondylitis, radial head or capitellar arthritis, capitellar osteochondritis Dissecans, posterolateral plica syndrome, and posterior interosseous nerve compression. It is important for surgeons treating elbow pain to be adept at performing the pivot shift test and the additional clinical tests outlined in this article to help distinguish PLRI from other causes of lateral elbow pain. We believe PLRI may be an initiating factor in the development of refractory lateral epicondylitis, and should be considered as one potential primary cause in this disorder.

The diagnosis is made by a combination of positive clinical findings supplemented by arthroscopic confirmation of instability. The posterolateral pivot shift test described by O'Driscoll and colleagues[1] can be performed both supine and prone, and combined with the interval rotation push-up and chair lift tests of Regan and Lapner,[5] to provide a clearer clinical picture of instability. These findings may coexist with the standard examination findings of lateral epicondylitis, radial tunnel, and posterolateral plica syndrome.

Additionally, the data suggest that the close proximity of the extensor carpi radialis brevis to the radial ulnohumeral ligament and LCL complex during lateral epicondylitis procedures may potentially contribute to the iatrogenic development of PLRI. The treating surgeon must carefully remain on the anterior border of the lateral epicondyle and avoid the inferior and posterior areas to avoid damage to the RUHL when performing a tennis elbow procedure.

Although in most series, repair seems to be an effective method of managing the instability, one should always be prepared to use a supplemental graft. We have found the number of previous surgeries and the time from the initial injury to definitive treatment to be the best predictors of the need for a graft.

SUMMARY

We have summarized 4 clinical tests for PL instability: (1) supine pivot shift, (2) prone pivot shift, (3) internal rotation wall push-up, and (4) chair push-up. We have also described an arthroscopic finding, the "elbow drive-through" sign, present in all patients with PL instability. Finally, we described both a ligament plication technique and a ligament repair technique that can be performed arthroscopically with a high rate of success as compared with open controls.

We believe that arthroscopic repair/plication of the RUHL can effectively repair PLRI. This article demonstrates that the described arthroscopic technique can be equally effective in achieving resolution of instability symptoms and offers a high degree of patient satisfaction.

REFERENCES

1. O'Driscoll SW, Bell DF, Morrey BF. Posterolateral rotatory instability of the elbow. J Bone Joint Surg Am 1991;73(3):440–6.

2. Dunning CE, Zarzour ZD, Patterson SD, et al. Ligamentous stabilizers against posterolateral rotator instability of the elbow. J Bone Joint Surg Am 2001; 83(12):1823–8.
3. Seki A, Olsen BS, Jensen SL, et al. Functional anatomy of the lateral collateral ligament complex of the elbow: configuration of Y and its role. J Shoulder Elbow Surg 2002;11(1):53–9.
4. Smith JP, Savoie FH, Field LD. Posterolateral rotatory instability of the elbow. Clin Sports Med 2001;20(1):47–58.
5. Regan W, Lapner PC. Prospective evaluation of two diagnostic apprehension signs for posterolateral instability of the elbow. J Shoulder Elbow Surg 2006; 15(3):344–6.
6. Potter HG, Weiland AJ, Schatz JA, et al. Posterolateral rotator instability of the elbow: usefulness of MR imaging in diagnosis. Radiology 1997;204:185–9.
7. Yadao MA, Savoie FH, Field LD. Posterolateral rotatory instability of the elbow. Instr Course Lect 2004;53:607–14.
8. Savoie FH, Field LD, Gurley DJ. Arthroscopic and open radial ulnohumeral ligament reconstruction for posterolateral rotatory instability of the elbow. In: Savoie FH, Field LD, editors. AANA Advanced Arthroscopy: The Elbow and Wrist. Saunders/Elsevier; 2010. p. 94–100.
9. Andrews JR, Carson WG. Arthroscopy of the elbow. Arthroscopy 1985;1(2): 97–107.
10. Kalainov DM, Cohen MS. Posterolateral rotatory instability of the elbow in association with lateral epicondylitis. A report of three cases. J Bone Joint Surg Am 2005;87(5):1120–5.

Ulnar Collateral Ligament Injury in the Overhead Athlete

Sanaz Hariri, MD[a], Marc R. Safran, MD[b],*

KEYWORDS

- Ulnar collateral ligament • Medial collateral ligament
- Valgus instability • Thrower's elbow • Throwing injuries
- Pitcher

Acute or chronic ulnar collateral ligament (UCL, also known as the medial collateral ligament) disruption or attenuation may cause medial elbow pain and valgus instability. In a 1941 description of shoulder and elbow injuries in professional baseball players, Bennett[1,2] described "a distinctive lesion" "not seen in other occupations": ossicles in the UCL that he attributed to chronic strain on the ligament. Waris[3] was the first to describe injury of the UCL in his 1946 description of isolated anterior oblique ligament (AOL) disruptions in javelin throwers. Even so, in 1981, Andrews[4] pointed out that "acute tears of the elbow's medial compartment have received little attention in orthopaedic literature" and attributed this omission to the observation that "the method of diagnosing instability in the acute condition is not widely known."

In the last quarter of a century, greater understanding of UCL anatomy and pathology, better diagnostic modalities, and heightened awareness of this injury has attracted greater interest in UCL injuries. UCL injuries are most common in athletes participating in overhead sports, such as baseball (especially pitchers), tennis, water polo, volleyball, golf, track and field (especially javelin), and football (especially the quarterback). UCL injury results in valgus instability, which may then predispose the athlete to disabling secondary elbow conditions (eg, ulnar neuritis; valgus extension overload syndrome affecting the posteromedial olecranon, the olecranon fossa, and the radiocapitellar joint; and potential generation of intra-articular loose bodies from the lateral and posterior compartments). This article reviews the functional anatomy and biomechanics of the UCL, the pathophysiology of the thrower's elbow, and its history, physical examination, imaging modalities, and treatment options.[5–7]

Funding support: none.
[a] Sports Medicine, Department of Orthopaedic Surgery, Stanford University, 1169 Trinity Drive, Menlo Park, CA 94025, USA
[b] Sports Medicine, Department of Orthopaedic Surgery, Stanford University, 450 Broadway Street, M/C 6342, Redwood City, CA 94063, USA
* Corresponding author.
E-mail address: msafran@stanford.edu

FUNCTIONAL ANATOMY

The UCL is a complex consisting of the AOL, the posterior oblique ligament (POL), and the transverse ligament (ligament of Cooper) (**Fig. 1**). The AOL originates on the flat portion of the anterior and inferior aspect of the medial epicondyle just posterior to the elbow axis (mean footprint 46 mm²) and inserts onto the sublime tubercle (the most prominent part of the medial ulnar tubercle, mean footprint 128 mm²), with a long tapered insertion running down the proximal medial ulna.[8,9] The mean length of the AOL is 27 mm and the mean width is 5 to 8 mm.[10–12] It is the strongest and stiffest elbow collateral ligament, with an average failure load of 260 N.[13] The AOL does not contain isometric fibers. However, nearly isometric areas are located on the lateral aspect of its medial epicondyle origin, having implications for reconstruction techniques.[14]

The POL is a fan-shaped ligament that is best defined when the elbow is flexed to approximately 90°. It originates from the medial epicondyle just posterior to the AOL origin and inserts along the base of the medial ulna's greater sigmoid notch. The mean length of the POL is 24 mm and the mean width is 5 to 8 mm (widest at its ulnar insertion).[11,12] The transverse ligament spans the insertion of the AOL and POL along the medial ulna, extending from the inferior medial coronoid process to the medial tip of the olecranon.[15,16]

Grossly, the AOL is the most discrete component of the UCL complex (ie, clearly distinguishable from the medial joint capsule), correlating to its histology. The AOL consists of 2 histologic layers: (1) distinct collagen bundles within the layers of the medial joint capsule, and (2) an additional ligament complex superficial to the capsular layers. The POL has just 1 layer: distinct collagen bundles within the layers of the medial joint capsule.[12]

FUNCTIONAL BIOMECHANICS

Overall, the UCL is the primary static elbow stabilizer to valgus stress.[17] Maximum valgus instability with transection of the UCL is present at 60° flexion.[18] In full extension, the UCL, anterior capsule, and bony articulation contribute equally to valgus stability; at 90° flexion, the anterior capsule relaxes and the UCL then contributes 54% of the valgus stabilizing force.[19] The AOL is the primary UCL contributor to valgus stability from 20° to 120° flexion.[20] The AOL is composed of an anterior band and posterior band that tighten in a reciprocal fashion as the elbow is flexed and extended. In the presence of valgus overload, the anterior band is most vulnerable in elbow extension, whereas the posterior band is more vulnerable in elbow flexion.[21]

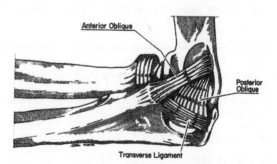

Fig. 1. Anatomy of the UCL complex. (*From* Safran MR. Elbow injuries in athletes. A review. Clin Orthop Relat Res 1995;310:257–77; with permission.)

The POL contributes to valgus stability to a greater degree as the elbow is flexed further; it is taut from 55° to 140° of elbow flexion. The transverse ligament does not seem to play a role in elbow stability because it connects 2 parts of the same bone and does not cross the joint.[15] The radiocapitellar articulation is a secondary valgus stabilizer. Although valgus instability does not arise when the radial head is resected in the presence of an intact UCL complex, a combined transection of the UCL and resection of the radial head results in gross valgus instability and subluxation.[22] Furthermore, injury to the UCL complex results in increased compressive forces at the radiocapitellar joint when a valgus force is applied.

The role of the olecranon-trochlear articulation in static valgus stability is controversial. There may be a reciprocal relationship: UCL insufficiently increases posteromedial compartment contact pressures at 30° elbow flexion, perhaps contributing to the development of posteromedial osteophytes.[23] Conversely, removal of the osteophytes and portions of the olecranon may destabilize the joint, placing more strain on the UCL. Andrews and Timmerman[24] reported that 5 of 34 baseball players who had an arthroscopic debridement of posterior olecranon osteophytes subsequently required UCL reconstruction for valgus instability. The investigators hypothesized that the absence of the posteromedial buttress could have destabilized the joint. Although it is likely that the UCL was injured before the index procedure in some of these athletes, the removal of part of the ulna could have placed further stress on the ligament.[24] In some biomechanical studies, valgus instability increases with sequential partial resection of the posteromedial aspect of the olecranon.[25,26] In one study, resection of more than 3 mm of the posteromedial olecranon jeopardized the function of the AOL.[27] However, a couple studies have reported that up to 8- to 12-mm posterior olecranon resection did not significantly affect UCL strain in a cadaver model.[28,29]

The forearm flexor tendons are the primary dynamic stabilizers to valgus stress. There is debate as to whether the flexor carpi ulnaris (FCU, which lies directly over the UCL) or the flexor digitorum superficialis (FDS, which lies near the UCL and has a large bulk) is the primary elbow dynamic stabilizer.[30–32] The flexor carpi radialis also contributes, but the pronator teres makes little, if any, contribution to valgus stability.[33] The flexor muscles (particularly the FDS) are histologically confluent with the underlying AOL fibers.[12] Even so, the contribution of the AOL to valgus stability is more than double that of the medial muscles.[34]

A description of the intricacies of elbow biomechanics,[15] upper extremity kinetic chain of force,[35] and biomechanical stresses on the elbow during various throwing motions (eg, a baseball pitch or football pass)[36] is beyond the scope of this article but is well detailed elsewhere.

PATHOPHYSIOLOGY OF THE THROWER'S ELBOW

Athletes engaging in repetitive high-velocity overhead motions (eg, baseball pitch, tennis serve, football pass, volleyball spike) and other motions involving significant valgus stress (eg, tennis forehands, golfing, hockey slap shots) experience (1) traction/tensile forces on their medial structures (ie, UCL, ulnar nerve, flexor-pronator mass), (2) compression forces on their lateral structures (ie, the radiocapitellar joint), and (3) compression/impingement forces in their posteromedial compartment. This article focuses on UCL injuries in the skeletally mature athlete.

The valgus force on the athlete's elbow can be significant. During a tennis serve, a maximum varus torque of approximately 68 N m is generated.[37] During a baseball pitch, the elbow generates a maximum varus torque (to counteract the valgus stress) of about 64 N m near the end of the arm cocking phase, but the UCL itself can only resist approximately 34 N m of torque before failing. The osseous anatomy, long axis rotation, contributions from the dynamic stabilizers, and other medial structures clearly assist in creating this counteracting varus torque.[38,39]

In pitching, maximum pitch velocity is significantly associated with risk of elbow injury. In one study, the pitchers with the highest maximum ball velocity were the ones who required surgery for UCL injuries.[40] Late trunk rotation, reduced shoulder external rotation, increased elbow flexion, and overhand pitching (vs side-arm delivery) are associated with reduced elbow valgus torque.[41] The parameters of pitching mechanics may therefore be accordingly modified to decrease the magnitude of valgus stress on the elbow.[42] Furthermore, the mechanics of tennis serve and volleyball spiking are more over the top, with the shoulder in greater degrees of abduction, resulting in decreased elbow valgus forces compared with baseball pitching, explaining the greater prevalence of these injuries in baseball.

Studies of youth pitchers have found that pitch count during a game, and cumulatively over a season, are significantly associated with elbow injuries.[43–45] Studying youth baseball pitchers, Dun and colleagues reported that the greatest mean varus torque is produced by the fastball (mean 35 N m), followed by the curveball (mean 32 N m), and then the change-up (mean 29 N m). The fastball torque is significantly greater than the curveball and change-up; the curveball torque is significantly greater than the change-up.[46] Lyman and colleagues studied the curveball, the change-up, and the slider and found that only the slider was associated with elbow pain, particularly in the 13 to 14 year olds.[43] In the collegiate pitcher, the greatest mean varus torque is produced by the fastball (mean 82 N m), followed by the slider (mean 81 N m), then the curveball (mean 79 N m), and then the change-up (mean 71 N m). The only significant differences were between the fastball versus the change-up and the curveball versus the change-up.[47] However, the rate of loading and the effect of forearm rotation with the curveball and slider may affect the forces on the UCL and medial elbow structures.

Chronic traction forces on the UCL may thicken the ligament and/or result in traction osteophytes at its insertion on the ulna. Repetitive valgus stresses can fatigue the flexor-pronator muscle mass (ie, the primary dynamic stabilizer to valgus stress), exposing the UCL to added stress and potentially hastening UCL attenuation/microtears, stretching, and eventual rupture.[48] In a study of 68 athletes with UCL tears, Conway and colleagues[49] reported the following UCL injury tear patterns: 87% torn at the midsubstance, 10% avulsed distally from the ulna, and 3% avulsed proximally from the medial epicondyle.

Stresses on the medial elbow can also lead to medial epicondylitis in these athletes. Reciprocally, stretching or rupture of the UCL exposes the medial dynamic stabilizers to added stress, hastening injury to those structures. This agonistic relationship is underscored by the finding of proximal flexor-pronator tendon partial tears in association with UCL tears. Norwood and colleagues[4] found concomitant proximal flexor-pronator tearing in all 4 of their operative UCL patients, and Conway and colleagues[49] reported a 13% incidence of proximal flexor-pronator mass tearing in their patients having UCL operations. More recently, in a study performed by Altchek of UCL reconstructions in baseball players, 4% had combined UCL and flexor-pronator injury. Age greater than 30 years was a significant predictor of this combined injury: only 1% of the isolated UCL patients were older than 30 years, whereas 7 of the 8 patients with combined flexor-pronator and UCL injuries were older than 30 years.[50]

There are several other elbow pathologies associated with UCL injuries. Valgus forces may cause traction neuritis of the ulnar nerve, which can be exacerbated by an incompetent UCL.[51–57] Furthermore, many baseball players have increased cubitus valgus in addition to flexion contractures, which places greater strain on the UCL. Chronic UCL injuries also lead to thickening and calcifications of the UCL, which is the floor of the cubital tunnel. Marginal osteophytes at the medial joint may develop from traction on the UCL. Posteromedial olecranon osteophytes may develop because of valgus extension overload. All of these anatomic changes contribute to a compressive, irritable environment for the ulnar nerve at the elbow.

Valgus torque leads to lateral elbow compressive forces of approximately 500 N between the radial head and humeral capitellum that is exacerbated by UCL laxity, potentially leading to avascular necrosis, osteochondritis dissecans, chondral wear, or osteochondral chip fractures.[38,58,59] The posteromedial elbow is compromised because traction osteophytes on the olecranon and hypertrophy of the distal humerus (which decreases the size of the olecranon fossa) results in repetitive posteromedial impingement, potentially leading to osteophytes, chondromalacia, and/or loose bodies.[38,60–64]

Immature athletes with open physes differ from adult athletes because their medial epicondylar apophysis is the weakest link on the medial side of the elbow. Repetitive valgus stresses and tension overload of medial structures may result in Little League elbow, a general term encompassing medial epicondylar avulsion, medial epicondylar apophysitis, and accelerated apophyseal growth with delayed closure of the epicondylar growth plate. Furthermore, the medial epicondyle (ie, the UCL origin) has a mildly forgiving attachment to the humerus via its physis. With valgus stress, the flexibility of the physis allows for increased elbow valgus, increasing the radiocapitellar load and potentially leading to osteochondritis dissecans. UCL injuries are uncommon in the skeletally immature athlete, but seem to be more frequently recognized of late.[65,66]

HISTORY

The athlete's age, sport, level of participation, hand dominance, laterality of the injury, and sports participation calendar (increasingly year-round) must be ascertained. Sports that predispose athletes to UCL injury include: baseball (especially pitchers), water polo, volleyball, tennis, golf, wrestling, arm wrestling, hockey, gymnastics, football (especially quarterbacks), and javelin throwing. In baseball, pitchers and catchers are more likely to sustain UCL injuries than infielders. UCL injuries are more common in high school and collegiate players than junior high players.[67] A history of previous elbow injuries, injections, bracing, and/or surgeries should be elicited.

For the throwing athlete, pertinent questions include the style of throwing mechanics, ball velocity before and after the onset of elbow pain, throwing accuracy, and phase(s) of throwing in which symptoms occur. Athletes most commonly report pain during the late-cocking or early acceleration phase of a throw; the point of ball/javelin release or when the racquet hits the ball is the second most common point of elbow pain.[49] Specific questions for the baseball pitcher include the types of pitches used, pitch counts, number of innings pitched, frequency of pitching, and the types of pitches that cause pain. Many structures contribute to the kinetic chain of throwing, and therefore a history of pain, injury, and/or surgery of more proximal structures (eg, ipsilateral shoulder, back, hip, knee, and/or ankle) is relevant.[35]

UCL injuries can be acute, chronic, or acute on chronic. A history of acute traumatic events affecting the elbow should be elicited. Those with an acute UCL rupture typically describe sudden onset of pain, often accompanied by a popping sensation, during a particular throw. Some recount an inability to throw after the injury. Overuse (eg, year-round pitching with high pitch counts) can cause chronic valgus instability caused by attenuation or complete rupture of the UCL. Athletes describe gradual onset of medial elbow soreness or pain with throwing, particularly in the late-cocking and acceleration phases. They may describe decreased velocity (eg, loss of zip or pop on the ball), distance, and accuracy of their pass or throw. They may note recurrent episodes of elbow pain that resolves with conservative management. Those with chronic valgus instability may also describe a sudden episode of giving way or severe elbow pain, likely representing rupture of a previously attenuated UCL. Athletes with chronic UCL injuries can often throw, but typically achieve no more than 60% to 80% of their preinjury maximal velocity.

A history of associated elbow pathologies must also be investigated. For example, loose bodies may present with mechanical symptoms (eg, catching or locking). Ulnar neuritis symptoms may include medial elbow pain radiating down the ulnar side of the forearm to the hand and numbness/tingling in the ulnar 2 digits. Athletes in particular may note clumsiness or heaviness of the hand and fingers associated with, and often exacerbated by, throwing or overhead activities. Ulnar neuritis can occur in both acute and chronic UCL injuries. In acute injuries, the nerve may be irritated by hemorrhage and edema. In chronic injuries, valgus instability subjects the ulnar nerve to higher tensile stresses, and there may be decreased space in the cubital tunnel because of UCL scarring. Symptoms may at first only occur with activity but, in time, may persist even with rest.

PHYSICAL EXAMINATION

The height and weight of the athlete should be noted; UCL injuries have been found to be more common in taller and heavier baseball players at the high school and collegiate level.[67] This may be because taller heavier players may throw harder and may therefore be more successful, thus they may be pitching more frequently and thus are more susceptible to overuse injuries. Alternatively, the taller player has longer extremities, resulting in a longer fulcrum and therefore greater forces on the UCL. During the physical examination, all maneuvers should be performed on both upper extremities for comparison. As with any joint, the examination should commence with inspection, palpation, and both active and passive motion of the upper extremities (including the shoulder, wrists, and hands). When the UCL is injured, the ipsilateral shoulder appears to have increased external rotation on physical examination.[68]

A thorough neurovascular examination should follow, with particular attention to the ulnar nerve distribution. The course of the UCL should be palpated. The UCL courses distal and slightly posterior to the medial epicondyle. Tenderness over the UCL has an 81% to 94% sensitivity but only a 22% specificity for UCL tears.[69,70] When there is an acute UCL injury, ecchymosis may develop along the medial elbow and proximal forearm 48 to 72 hours afterwards. The elbow should be assessed for a fixed flexion and valgus deformity, sometimes seen in older baseball pitchers, which can predispose athletes to ulnar neuritis.[71,72]

Examination of the shoulder and scapula is critical because altered mechanics proximally can alter throwing mechanics through the kinetic chain. A glenohumeral internal rotation deficit is associated with valgus instability in throwers.[73] Kibler recently showed that individuals with clinically significant UCL injuries have a higher prevalence of glenohumeral internal rotation deficits, scapular dyskinesis, and hip weakness and/or inflexibility (Kibler WB, personal communication, 2010). The neck should be assessed as a potential source of referred pain. The presence or absence of a palmaris longus (PL) tendon should be noted (ask the patient to touch the ipsilateral thumb and small finger and flex the wrist to detect the tendon) because this is a potential autograft source for UCL reconstruction. The PL is absent in 1 extremity in 3% and absent in both extremities in 2.5% of white people in North America.[74]

The diagnosis of medial epicondylitis must be considered, although the presence of medial epicondylitis does not rule out UCL injury because they may coexist. Patients with flexor-pronator epicondylitis have pain with resisted wrist flexion when the elbow is fully extended and localize their pain just anterior and distal to the common flexor muscle origin. In contrast, patients with a UCL injury typically have point tenderness about 2 cm distal to their medial epicondyle. Concomitant flexor-pronator tearing presents with tenderness over the medial epicondylar muscle origin and pain and weakness elicited with resisted wrist flexion with the elbow fully extended.

The most critical component of the physical examination when UCL injury is suspected is assessment of the UCL functional integrity through various tests subjecting the elbow to a valgus force and assessing for medial joint space opening, the quality of the end point (if it exists), and medial-sided pain. The center of the elbow varus-valgus axis is along the center of the trochlea, which is located medial to the midline. Therefore, valgus elbow stress with compromised medial structures produces less medial gapping than varus stress when the lateral structures are injured. The medial joint space opens only a few millimeters even with a complete UCL rupture, making detection of valgus instability by physical examination difficult and heightening the importance of comparing findings with the contralateral side. Accordingly, even the most experienced elbow surgeons are only able to detect preoperative valgus laxity on physical examination in between 26%[75] and 82%[69] of patients with operative UCL tear.

Cadaver studies have sought to determine the optimal elbow flexion and forearm rotation for detecting valgus instability in an elbow with a compromised or torn UCL. There are no significant differences in valgus laxity with respect to elbow flexion when comparing 30°, 50°, and 70° of elbow flexion, because the contributions of the anterior capsular and bony contributions are minimized in this range. However, testing in forearm-neutral rotation elicits the greatest valgus instability.[76]

Traditionally, in the elbow abduction stress test, the humerus is stabilized and the elbow is subjected to a valgus stress at about 20° to 30° elbow flexion (**Fig. 2**). In a positive test, there is no firm end point and the articular surfaces of the ulna and medial humeral condyle are felt to move apart and the forearm swings out laterally.[4] About half of patients with a torn UCL report pain with valgus stress testing.[69] This

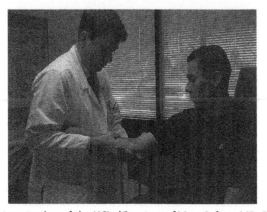

Fig. 2. Abduction stress testing of the UCL. (*Courtesy of* Marc Safran, MD, Redwood City, CA.)

test is 66% sensitive and 60% specific for detecting abnormalities of the anterior band of the AOL.[70] The milking maneuver, testing the posterior band of the AOL, involves generating a valgus force by pulling the patient's thumb with the patient's forearm supinated, shoulder extended, and elbow flexed beyond 90°. Patients with a UCL injury may report a feeling of apprehension, instability, and medial joint pain.[55]

The senior author prefers a modification of the milking maneuver. The arm being tested is in shoulder adduction and maximum external rotation, removing shoulder external rotation as a confounding variable. The examiner uses one hand to position the elbow being tested in 70° of flexion with the examiner's thumb on the medial joint line (**Fig. 3**) (70°of elbow flexion was identified in a cadaver study to be the position of greatest valgus laxity when the UCL is sectioned).[18] The examiner's other hand is used to pull down on the patient's thumb on the arm being examined, creating a valgus stress. The examiner's hand that is being used to hold the elbow is also used to palpate the medial joint line to feel for joint space opening and an end point.

To perform the moving valgus stress test as described by O'Driscoll and colleagues,[77] the patient's shoulder is held in 90° of abduction and external rotation. The examiner applies and maintains a constant moderate valgus torque to the fully flexed elbow and then quickly extends the elbow. In a positive test, the patient complains of maximal medial elbow pain between 120° and 70° of elbow flexion (**Fig. 4**). There is 100% sensitivity and 75% specificity using arthroscopic valgus stress testing and surgical exploration of the UCL as the gold standard.[77]

DIAGNOSIS: IMAGING AND ARTHROSCOPY

Several imaging modalities may be useful in elucidating various nuances in UCL injury, aiding in the diagnosis and helping guide the choice of treatment. Plain radiographs may reveal an avulsion fragment in an acute injury. In chronic UCL injuries, ossification of the UCL, loose bodies, and radiocapitellar and/or ulnohumeral osteophytes may be seen (**Fig. 5**). In a population of patients who had surgery for elbow pain, 76% of those

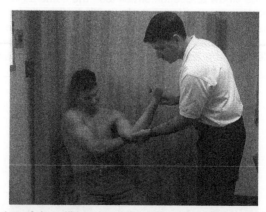

Fig. 3. A modification of the milking maneuver. The patient adducts and externally rotates the arm/shoulder to be examined. The examiner places a hand on the elbow to be examined; that hand is used to stabilize the elbow and to palpate the medial joint line for medial joint gapping and for the quality of the end point. The patient flexes the elbow being examined to 70° and the examiner imparts a valgus stress by pulling down on the ipsilateral thumb. The examiner assesses medial joint laxity (gapping) and quality of end point and notes pain with valgus stress. The test is repeated on the contralateral elbow for comparison. (*Courtesy of* Marc Safran, MD, Redwood City, CA.)

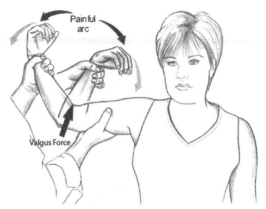

Fig. 4. The moving valgus stress test as described by O'Driscoll and colleagues.[77] The shoulder is abducted and externally rotated. The examiner applies and maintains a constant moderate valgus torque to the fully flexed elbow and then quickly extends the elbow. In a positive test, the patient complains of maximal medial elbow pain between 120° and 70° of elbow flexion. (*Courtesy of* Marc Safran, MD, Redwood City, CA.)

with heterotopic calcification of the UCL evident on plain radiographs were found to have either partial or complete tears of the UCL.[78]

Stress radiographs can be used to detect increased ulnohumeral gapping with valgus stress in the injured elbow compared with the uninjured elbow (**Fig. 6**).

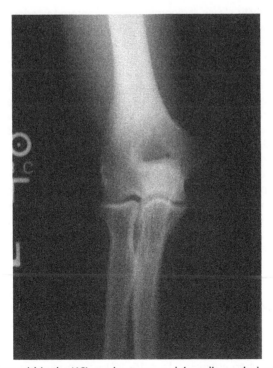

Fig. 5. Calcifications within the UCL can be seen on plain radiographs in chronic injuries, as seen with this 22-year-old professional baseball player. (*Courtesy of* Marc Safran, MD, Redwood City, CA.)

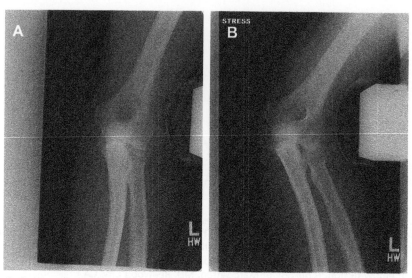

Fig. 6. Stress radiography: 21-year-old collegiate javelin thrower with elbow pain. (*A*) The elbow without stress applied, demonstrating calcification within the UCL. (*B*) The elbow with a valgus force applied using a valgus stress device. (*Courtesy of* Marc Safran, MD, Redwood City, CA.)

Historically, the gravity stress radiograph was an anteroposterior radiograph of the elbow performed with the patient supine, the shoulder in maximum external rotation, and the forearm unsupported so that the elbow is essentially parallel to the floor. Another technique had the examiner apply a valgus load to the elbow while the anteroposterior radiograph was obtained. The problem with the former technique was that there may not be enough valgus torque applied, whereas the problem with both of these techniques is there is likely an inconsistent amount of elbow flexion and differing degrees of humeral and/or forearm rotation affecting measurements of ulnohumeral gapping. With the manual stress test, the amount of force applied to the 2 elbows was not controlled, and thus may differ. Alternatively, a device that applies a uniform valgus stress may be used to obtain a stress radiograph to assess medial joint space widening compared with the contralateral elbow.[69,75,79] These devices ensure a uniform force applied with consistent elbow flexion and rotation. However, the senior author has not found these devices to be sufficiently sensitive in detecting UCL laxity.[80]

Field and Altchek[81] studied the magnitude of medial gapping based on UCL injury pattern in cadavers. There was no gapping visible on elbow arthroscopy until the AOL was completely sectioned, yielding 1 to 2 mm of joint opening. Dramatic gapping (4–10 mm) only occurred after complete sectioning of the UCL (transection of both the AOL and POL). Maximal gapping occurred at 60° to 70° of elbow flexion.[81]

The comparison of medial gapping between the dominant and nondominant elbow differs depending on the study population. In the general, uninjured population, there is no difference in medial gapping as a result of valgus stress between the 2 elbows of an individual.[82] In contrast, even at baseline, the medial joint space of an uninjured professional pitcher's dominant elbow opens up a significantly greater distance (1.20 ± 0.97 mm) when subjected to a 15-daN valgus stress compared with their nondominant elbow (0.88 ± 0.55 mm).[79] One study found that, in an athlete, joint space widening on stress radiographs (15 daN applied) of greater than 0.5 mm in the affected elbow compared with the opposite normal elbow indicated a significant partial tear or a complete tear of the UCL. Athletes with widening less than 0.5 mm on stress radiographs compared with the normal elbow had a normal UCL or just a small tear that could be managed conservatively.[83]

Azar and colleagues[75] reported that 46% of their UCL reconstruction athletes had positive preoperative valgus stress views. Thompson and colleagues[69] reported that 88% of their athletes having UCL reconstruction had greater than 2 mm of opening to valgus stress before their operations compared with the contralateral elbow on stress radiographs.

An arthrogram is particularly useful in an acute UCL injury when the medial capsule may be ruptured, visualized as contrast leakage from the joint. Arthrography is also helpful in detecting partial undersurface tearing of the UCL, creating a T sign in which the dye leaks around the detachment of the UCL from its bony insertion but remains contained within the joint by the intact superficial layer of the UCL (**Fig. 7**).[70,84]

Computed tomography (CT) arthrograms are 71% to 86% sensitive and 91% specific for UCL tears.[70,75] Magnetic resonance imaging (MRI) is 57% to 79% sensitive and 100% specific for UCL tears.[69,70] A magnetic resonance (MR) arthrogram is 97% sensitive for UCL tears and is the senior author's study of choice to evaluate the patient with suspected UCL tear after plain radiographs are obtained.[75] UCL injury may present on MRI as ligament laxity, irregularity, poor definition, and increased signal intensity within and adjacent to the ligament because of hemorrhage and/or edema. The UCL fibers are disrupted in complete tears; fluid extravasation is evident on MR arthrograms (**Figs. 8** and **9**).[85,86] Associated injuries, such as damage to the articular cartilage of the trochlea and olecranon fossa, subchondral edema of the radiocapitellar joint, tearing or inflammation of the common flexor origin, and inflammation of the ulnar nerve, can also be seen on MRI.[87]

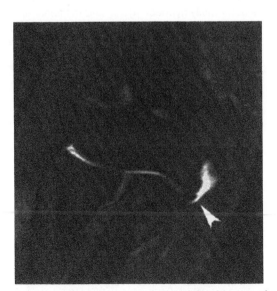

Fig. 7. Magnetic resonance arthrogram: coronal T2-weighted image of a partial-thickness undersurface tear of the UCL in an 18-year-old collegiate softball player. Fluid outlines the tear (T sign) but does not extravasate as the superficial UCL is still intact. (*Courtesy of* Marc Safran, MD, Redwood City, CA.)

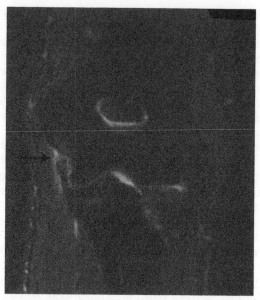

Fig. 8. MRI: coronal T2-weighted image of a proximal full-thickness tear of the UCL in a 20-year-old wrestler. (*Courtesy of* Marc Safran, MD, Redwood City, CA.)

Ultrasonography (US) is a rapid UCL evaluation modality; both elbows can be examined in an average of just more than 10 minutes. In a cadaver study, a normal UCL has a compact fibrillar echotexture and appears hyperechoic between the medial epicondyle and proximal ulna. The proximal UCL varies from a cordlike structure to a broad attachment to the undersurface of the medial epicondyle, with variable surrounding fat. Injured UCLs are abnormally hypoechogenic and the fibers appear disrupted.[88,89] In pitching arms of professional baseball players, the AOL is thicker, more likely to have hypoechoic foci and/or calcifications, and has more laxity with valgus stress

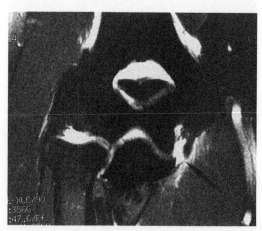

Fig. 9. MR arthrogram: coronal T2-weighted image of a distal full-thickness tear of the UCL in a 25-year-old baseball player. Note the lateral fluid extravasation. (*Courtesy of* Marc Safran, MD, Redwood City, CA.)

than the nonpitching arm.[90] When the UCL is ruptured, US reveals discontinuity of the normally hyperechoic ligament with anechoic fluid in the gap or nonvisualization of the ligament with heterogeneous echogenicity in the expected location of the ligament. When the UCL is sprained, US may show thickening, decreased echogenicity of the ligament, and surrounding hypoechoic edema compared with the contralateral normal elbow.[91] Ciccotti[92] followed 155 professional athletes on whom he had performed dynamic US over 6 years. According to his preliminary data, athletes who sustained a UCL tear had preinjury joint space gapping of more than 1 to 1.5 mm on valgus stress and had UCL calcifications before the injury.[92]

Dynamic US can demonstrate medial joint instability by comparing the ulnotrochlear joint width of the elbows when subject to valgus stress.[93] However, at baseline, the medial joint space is significantly wider on the throwing, compared with the nonthrowing, elbow in baseball players (2.7 mm and 1.6 mm, respectively, with gravity valgus stress).[94]

The role of arthroscopy in evaluating valgus instability has been studied. The ulnohumeral joint is viewed through the anterolateral portal. Partial and full-thickness tears of the UCL can be diagnosed by arthroscopically visualizing the magnitude of medial joint gapping: 1 to 2 mm for partial tears (just the AOL) and 4 to 10 mm for complete tears. Visualization of the medial joint opening is best at 60° to 75° of elbow flexion with the forearm pronated.[81] Timmerman and colleagues[70] found that all patients with valgus instability on arthroscopic testing had AOL pathology, and all those without valgus instability on arthroscopic testing had an intact and normal AOL on surgical exploration.

TREATMENT
Nonoperative

UCL injuries are initially treated with rest, antiinflammatory medications (nonsteroidal antiinflammatory drugs [NSAIDs]), bracing, and/or physical therapy. Rettig and colleagues[95] described a 2-phase rehabilitation protocol. The first 2 to 3 months consists of no throwing, NSAIDs, icing for 10 minutes 4 times a day, splint/brace at 90° at night and as needed for pain during the day, and active and passive range of motion exercises for flexors and pronators. If patients are pain free at the end of the first phase, they can then discontinue the splint/brace, start progressive upper extremity strengthening program of all muscle groups, begin a throwing progression at 3 months, and use an elbow hyperextension brace for throwing and lifting. Forty-two percent of their throwing athletes were able to return to their previous levels of competition at an average of 24.5 weeks after diagnosis. They could not identify a component of the history or physical examination that predicted the success of nonoperative treatment.[95]

Repair

Surgical treatment of UCL partial and complete tears has evolved, and is continuing to evolve, over time. In 1980, Schwab and colleagues[20] described a treatment to tighten the stretched, incompetent UCL: osteotomy of the medial humeral epicondyle including the proximal origin of the UCL, transfer of the fragment proximal and volar, and fixation with a screw. This technique is no longer used because the attenuated ligament is believed to have been weakened by repeated microtrauma, the transferred position is not isometric, and a resultant flexion contracture may not be acceptable in a high-level athlete.

Primary UCL repair is an option when adequate, normal-appearing UCL tissue remains. When there is an avulsion injury off the bone, the UCL can be repaired by direct suture fixation, sutures using drill holes, or suture anchors. Midsubstance tears can be repaired end to end or imbricated.[4,49,96] Conway and colleagues[49] reported their results in 14 cases: 7 excellent, 3 good, 2 fair, and 2 poor. However, only 2 of their 7 Major League baseball (MLB) players returned to MLB after a repair, compared with 12 of 16 after primary reconstructions. Similarly, Azar and colleagues[75] reported better return to previous or higher levels of competition in their reconstruction group compared with the repair group (81% vs 63%).

Consequently, direct repair is now only advocated for the following patient population: acute injury, no ulnar nerve symptoms, operation performed soon after injury, and the UCL appears normal except for complete separation from bone.[49] Richard and colleagues[97,98] reported on the direct repair of acute traumatic UCL ruptures from the humerus using bone tunnels or suture anchors at a mean 20 days from the date of injury. All patients were found to have an avulsed flexor-pronator tendon with distal retraction, which was repaired using interrupted figure-of-eight sutures. Nine of their 11 patients were able to return to competitive college athletics between 4 and 6 months after their operations.[97,98] Savoie and colleagues[99] focused on proximal and distal UCL avulsion injuries in young athletes (mean age 17 years) with the assumption that these patients would have less chronic damage to their ligaments. They repaired the avulsion using suture plication with repair to bone drill holes or suture repair to bone using anchors. Fifty-eight of their 60 patients returned to their sport at the same or higher level within 6 months of the surgery.[99] It may be that the younger athletes have more acute insertional injuries, whereas adults tend to have chronic intrasubstance damage.

Reconstruction

UCL reconstruction is now the surgery of choice for most acute and chronic UCL injuries. Indications for UCL reconstruction include (1) acute ruptures in high-level throwers, (2) significant chronic instability, (3) insufficient UCL tissue remaining after UCL debridement for calcifications, and (4) recurrent pain and subtle valgus instability with throwing after supervised rehabilitation.[5] In general, UCL reconstruction entails fixing a graft to bone through tunnel(s) in the humeral epicondyle and the ulnar sublime tubercle to reestablish valgus stability. Graft options include ipsilateral or contralateral PL, hamstring tendon, fourth toe extensor, plantaris tendon, strip of the Achilles tendon, or allograft (usually hamstring or posterior or anterior tibialis tendon).

Frank W. Jobe developed the original UCL reconstruction technique. He performed the first AOL reconstructive surgery on pitcher Tommy John in 1974; John proceeded to win 164 games after the procedure.[100] Jobe and colleagues[101] described transection of the common flexor-pronator tendon then reflection of the tendon and muscle distally to expose the injured UCL, a figure-of-eight graft weave through drill holes in the ulna and humerus, and submuscular ulnar nerve transposition (**Fig. 10**). They reported that 10 of the 16 athletes (63%) were able to return to their sport at the same level of competition.[101]

Numerous modifications to the Jobe technique have since been described.[102,103] Because the FCU and FDS are the primary dynamic stabilizers of the medial elbow, muscle-splitting techniques[69,104] and techniques elevating and retracting the flexor-pronator tendon anteriorly without detaching or splitting it[75] have been developed to decrease soft tissue morbidity. The ulnar nerve is no longer routinely transposed because up to 21% of patients can have postoperative neurologic problems with transposition.[49,104] Furthermore, instead of drilling the humeral tunnel posteriorly,

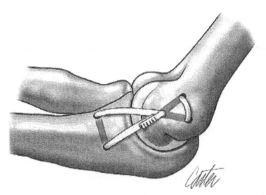

Fig. 10. The original figure-of-eight UCL reconstruction technique as developed by Jobe. (*From* Shah RP, Lindsey DP, Sungar GW, et al. An analysis of four ulnar collateral ligament reconstruction procedures with cyclic valgus loading. J Shoulder Elbow Surg 2009;18:59; with permission.)

the tunnel is now directed anteriorly to prevent penetration of the posterior cortex and to protect the ulnar nerve.[69]

The docking procedure was developed by David Altchek and described in 2002, involving docking the 2 ends of the tendon graft into a single blind-ended humeral tunnel and tying the sutures over a humeral bone bridge (**Fig. 11**). Rohrbough and colleagues[105] reported that 92% of the athletes returned to or exceeded their previous level of competition for at least 1 year. A cadaver study found that both the muscle-splitting Jobe technique and the docking technique provide valgus stability comparable to the native UCL at 90° to 110° flexion, the range in which peak valgus torque is experience in the throwing elbow. However, both provide less valgus stability than the native UCL at lower flexion angles, suggesting that motions such as side-arm throwing should be cautioned against after operations.[106] The senior author finds that tensioning the graft using the docking procedure is easier than the figure-of-eight technique.

Koh and colleagues[107] described a modified docking technique, using a 3-strand construct with a double anterior bundle and a single posterior bundle (**Fig. 12**). They

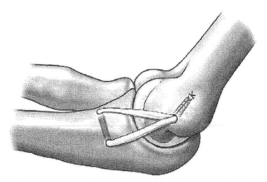

Fig. 11. The docking UCL reconstruction technique as developed by Altchek. The 2 ends of the tendon graft are docked into a single blind-ended humeral tunnel and the sutures are tied over a humeral bone bridge. (*From* Shah RP, Lindsey DP, Sungar GW, et al. An analysis of four ulnar collateral ligament reconstruction procedures with cyclic valgus loading. J Shoulder Elbow Surg 2009;18(1):60; with permission.)

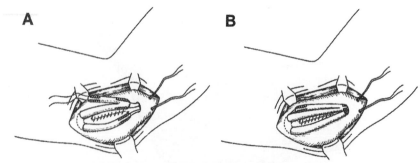

Fig. 12. A modified docking technique described by Koh and colleagues[107] using a 3-strand construct with a double anterior bundle and a single posterior bundle. (*From* Shah RP, Lindsey DP, Sungar GW, et al. An analysis of four ulnar collateral ligament reconstruction procedures with cyclic valgus loading. J Shoulder Elbow Surg 2009;18(1):58–63; with permission.)

reported excellent outcomes in 17 patients and a good outcome in 2; 18 of the 19 had returned to their previous level of participation or higher at a mean return-to-play time of 13.1 months.[107] Paletta and Wright[108] described their modified docking technique using a quadruple-stranded instead of a double-stranded PL. They reported that 92% of their athletes were able to return to their preinjury levels of competition at a mean of 11.5 months (range, 10–16 months) after their operations.[108] In a cadaver study, there was no significant difference between the maximal moment to failure between this modified docking construct and the native UCL; both were significantly higher than the Jobe construct.[109] Adding an interference screw into the humeral tunnel increases the stiffness of the construct and increases the moment needed to create a 3-mm medial joint space gap, but it does not increase the ultimate moment of failure.[110]

Techniques that decrease the technical difficulty and necessary exposure for reconstruction have been studied in cadavers, with encouraging biomechanical results, but clinical data are not yet available. For example, Ahmad and colleagues[39] described an interference screw reconstruction (ISR) technique, fixing the graft into a single tunnel in the medial epicondyle and a single tunnel in the sublime tubercle using soft tissue interference screws. The purported benefit of the interference screw technique is reduced surgical dissection, particularly at the ulna where only a single tunnel is necessary. Making just a single drill hole rather than 2 reduces the risks of ulnar nerve injury and tunnel blowout. They reported failure strength of the ISR comparable with that of the native ligament.[39] However, Large and colleagues[111] reported that the ISR technique was inferior to the traditional Jobe reconstruction in terms of failure strength and initial and overall stiffness. McAdams and colleagues[112] found that the ISR construct has less valgus angle widening in response to early cyclic valgus loading (10–100 cycles) compared with the docking technique, but there was no difference between the 2 constructs by the 1000th cycle.

The DANE TJ (named after David Altchek, Neal ElAttrache, and Tommy John) technique has been proposed and advocated particularly for revision cases and cases of sublime tubercle insufficiency. It is a hybrid technique using interference screw fixation on the ulnar side and docking technique fixation on the humeral side (**Fig. 13**).[113] Nineteen of their 22 patients had excellent results, 2 fair, and 1 poor (a revision case); 2 developed ulnar neuritis.[114]

There are several other recently published comparative biomechanical studies of modified UCL construction techniques, including EndoButton fixation at the ulnar tunnel[115]; an interference humeral knot using a semitendinosus graft[116]; an

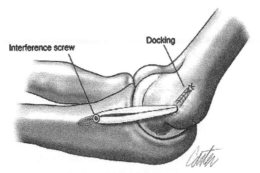

Fig. 13. The DANE TJ reconstruction technique: a hybrid of the David Altchek docking procedure on the humeral side and the Neal ElAttrache interference screw technique on the ulnar side. Tommy John is the pitcher on whom Jobe originally performed his figure-of-eight UCL reconstruction. (*From* Shah RP, Lindsey DP, Sungar GW, et al. An analysis of four ulnar collateral ligament reconstruction procedures with cyclic valgus loading. J Shoulder Elbow Surg 2009;18(1):60; with permission.)

arthroscopically assisted, all-interference screw transolecranon fossa ulnar collateral ligament reconstruction technique[117]; and suspension button fixation for the ulnar fixation in cases of ulnar cortical bone loss.[118] Hechtman and colleagues[119] compared the mean strengths of reconstruction using bone tunnels with bone anchors (76.3% vs 63.5% of normal elbow strength, respectively). There was no significant difference in reconstruction strength between the two, with the anchor being less invasive and less technically challenging. None of these modifications have published clinical results yet.

Rehabilitation After UCL Reconstruction

Focus on the athlete's body and throwing mechanics is critical to postoperative rehabilitation. One must not forget to maintain shoulder flexibility and strength (including the scapular stabilizers), as well as core strength. The senior author's preferred protocol is for the elbow to be initially splinted in 70° to 90° of flexion at neutral forearm rotation to allow skin and soft tissue healing. At the 10-day follow-up visit, the splint is removed and active wrist, elbow, and shoulder range of motion exercises are initiated, with a hinged elbow brace beginning at 30° to 100°. Range of motion is progressed such that there should be full range of motion by 6 weeks. At 4 to 6 weeks after the operation, the athlete is progressed to strengthening exercises that avoid elbow valgus stress. The elbow brace is removed at 8 weeks.

A recent biomechanical study sought to define safe rehabilitation for this initial postoperative period. They reported that movement between full extension and flexion of 50° is safe at any forearm rotation, but further flexion exceeded their safe-zone of less than 3% mean strains on the reconstruction. Isometric muscle contractions had no effect on strain.[120]

At 14 to 16 weeks, a throwing progression is initiated, beginning with ball toss of 9 to 12 m (30–40 feet) 2 to 3 times a week for about 15 minutes. This program is progressed such that the average pitcher returns to play at approximately 10 months. Position players return a month or two earlier. The protocol should be individualized to the athlete's sport.[5]

UCL Reconstruction Results and Results in the Female Athlete

UCL reconstruction has revolutionized the perception of UCL surgery. When he first described his technique in 1986, Jobe and colleagues[101] noted, "There was a widespread belief among the baseball pitchers that they would never again pitch competitively after undergoing a major operation on the elbow." A recent study revealed that 82% of pitchers return to Major League play at a mean of 18.5 months after the Tommy John surgery (ie, UCL reconstruction) without any significant changes in their mean earned run average or walks and hits per innings pitched. By the second season after injury, there was no difference between mean innings pitched between the reconstruction group and the control group (a random sampling of MLB pitchers).[100]

There are no randomized controlled studies assessing UCL reconstruction.[102] The recently developed Kerlan-Jobe Orthopaedic Clinic Overhead Athlete Shoulder and Elbow Score (KJOC score) is the most sensitive score for detecting subtle changes in performance in the throwing athlete and has been validated for evaluation of the overhead athlete undergoing UCL reconstruction.[121]

A recent systematic review of reconstruction methods attributed the muscle-splitting approach to the flexor-pronator mass, decreased handling of the ulnar nerve, and the use of the docking technique to the improved outcomes and reduced complication rates. They found a 76% rate of excellent results and 8% rate of postoperative ulnar neuropathy using the figure-of-eight technique, a 90% rate of excellent results and 3% rate of postoperative ulnar neuropathy using the docking technique, and a 95% rate of excellent results and 5% rate of postoperative ulnar neuropathy using the modified docking techniques.[122]

Andrews[123] presented the complications of UCL reconstruction in a series of more than 1200 UCL reconstruction cases with more than 2 years of follow-up. In terms of nerve complications, he noted that 6.4% experienced temporary ulnar paresthesias, 0.9% experienced major persistent ulnar sensory/motor symptoms (half resolved within a year and half required decompression), and 6% had damage to their medial antebrachial cutaneous nerve. There was a 2% retear rate, 4% lost more than 20° of extension (although 72% of them returned to play), a 4.9% rate of posterior impingement, a 1.8% risk of medial epicondylar fracture (risk: preoperative medial epicondylitis), 5% had nonspecific elbow pain (mostly young throwers), and 6% complained of graft site discomfort.[123]

Predictably, the rate of return to play is much lower, and the complication rate is higher, in revision UCL reconstruction compared with primary reconstruction. In a retrospective study of 15 revision cases, 11 were Jobe reconstructions, 3 DANE TJs, and 1 primary repair. Only 5 of the 15 returned to their previous level of play for at least 1 season (4 modified Jobes and 1 DANE TJ); other results included 4 good, 2 fair, and 4 poor (3 modified Jobes and 1 DANE TJ).[124]

Argo and colleagues[125] examined the results of operative treatment of UCL injuries in female athletes. Of the 19, 18 were athletes: 8 softball players (only 1 was a pitcher), 4 gymnasts, 2 tennis players, 1 snow skier, 1 calf roper, 1 cheerleader, and 1 baton twirler. Surgical treatment included repair of UCL to bone using anchors (11) or drill holes (1), plication (6), and palmaris graft reconstruction (1). Seventeen of the 18 athletes returned to their sport at a mean 2.5 months after their operations.[125]

Treatment of Associated Pathology

There are a few procedures that are often performed in conjunction with UCL repair or reconstruction for associated pathologies. Loose bodies can be removed arthroscopically.[126–128] Injury to the flexor-pronator mass (tendonitis, partial tearing, or avulsion) is associated with UCL tears. Altchek performed a docking procedure for the UCL and treated the flexor-pronator injury with debridement if tendinotic or reattachment if torn.

Outcomes were inferior to isolated UCL injuries: 1 excellent, 2 fair, and 5 poor. Only 13% returned to prior level of play.[50]

Posteromedial osteophytes can be removed from the olecranon in athletes who present with valgus extension overload. Athletes with posteromedial olecranon osteophytes should be carefully evaluated for UCL pathology because the same valgus forces generating those osteophytes also strain the UCL. As discussed earlier, Andrews and Timmerman[24] reported that 5 of 34 baseball players required UCL reconstruction for valgus instability after an arthroscopic debridement of posterior olecranon osteophytes. It is unclear whether the UCL pathology was simply overlooked initially or whether removal of the posteromedial buttress destabilized the joint, either stressing the UCL or unmasking underlying UCL damage; possibly a combination of these factors was at play.[24] When addressing these posteromedial olecranon osteophytes, the senior author recommends removal of just the osteophytes, leaving the normal olecranon intact to minimize destabilization of the joint.

SUMMARY

The UCL is the primary restraint to elbow valgus instability. Overhead throwing sports place significant stress on the UCL. Athletes may experience acute ruptures or avulsion of the UCL, or may have a progressively attenuated UCL caused by overuse. UCL injuries are associated with other elbow pathologies and may contribute to the development of these associated conditions via increased valgus instability: ulnar neuritis, valgus extension overload syndrome compromising the posterior compartment of the elbow and/or the radiocapitellar joint, and intra-articular loose bodies. Perhaps the most sensitive diagnostic modalities are the moving valgus stress test as described by O'Driscoll and colleagues,[77] the modified milking maneuver, and an MR arthrogram. For those less than 20 years of age, a primary repair may be considered, especially in cases of acute avulsion injuries. Otherwise UCL reconstruction using a graft (usually the PL) is now the standard of care for most UCL tears.

The Jobe figure-of-eight technique was the first reconstruction procedure. Modifications of the Altchek docking technique are now the most common reconstructions, offering a less invasive approach, lower chance of postoperative ulnar neuritis, and higher success rates. If the patient has a good-sized graft (either the PL or hamstring if the palmaris is absent), then the senior author's preferred procedure is the docking technique. If the graft is small, then the authors prefer the modified Jobe 3-ply figure-of-eight technique or obtaining an alternative graft. If there are no or minimal ulnar nerve symptoms, we prefer to use the muscle-splitting approach and leave the nerve intact. If there are significant ulnar nerve symptoms, then we prefer to perform a subcutaneous ulnar nerve transposition and to use the approach described by Andrews,[75] elevating the flexor-pronator mass. The prognosis for return to play at preinjury levels is now better than 90% following current reconstruction procedures.

REFERENCES

1. Bennett GE. Elbow and shoulder lesions of baseball players: George E. Bennett MD (1885–1962). The 8th president of the AAOS 1939. Clin Orthop Relat Res 2008;466(1):62–73.
2. Bennett GE. Shoulder and elbow lesions of the professional baseball pitcher. JAMA 1941;117:510–4.
3. Waris W. Elbow injuries in javelin throwers. Acta Chir Scand 1946;93:563–75.
4. Norwood LA, Shook JA, Andrews JR. Acute medial elbow ruptures. Am J Sports Med 1981;9(1):16–9.

5. Safran M, Ahmad CS, ElAttrache NS. Ulnar collateral ligament of the elbow. Arthroscopy 2005;21(11):1381–95.
6. Safran MR. Ulnar collateral ligament injury in the overhead athlete: diagnosis and treatment. Clin Sports Med 2004;23(4):643–63, x.
7. Safran MR. Elbow injuries in athletes. A review. Clin Orthop Relat Res 1995;310: 257–77.
8. O'Driscoll SW, Jaloszynski R, Morrey BF, et al. Origin of the medial ulnar collateral ligament. J Hand Surg Am 1992;17(1):164–8.
9. Dugas JR, Ostrander RV, Cain EL, et al. Anatomy of the anterior bundle of the ulnar collateral ligament. J Shoulder Elbow Surg 2007;16(5):657–60.
10. Cage DJ, Abrams RA, Callahan JJ, et al. Soft tissue attachments of the ulnar coronoid process. An anatomic study with radiographic correlation. Clin Orthop Relat Res 1995;320:154–8.
11. Morrey BF, An KN. Functional anatomy of the ligaments of the elbow. Clin Orthop Relat Res 1985;201:84–90.
12. Timmerman LA, Andrews JR. Histology and arthroscopic anatomy of the ulnar collateral ligament of the elbow. Am J Sports Med 1994;22(5):667–73.
13. Regan WD, Korinek SL, Morrey BF, et al. Biomechanical study of ligaments around the elbow joint. Clin Orthop Relat Res 1991;271:170–9.
14. Armstrong AD, Ferreira LM, Dunning CE, et al. The medial collateral ligament of the elbow is not isometric: an in vitro biomechanical study. Am J Sports Med 2004;32(1):85–90.
15. Alcid JG, Ahmad CS, Lee TQ. Elbow anatomy and structural biomechanics. Clin Sports Med 2004;23(4):503–17, vii.
16. Fuss FK. The ulnar collateral ligament of the human elbow joint. Anatomy, function and biomechanics. J Anat 1991;175:203–12.
17. Hotchkiss RN, Weiland AJ. Valgus stability of the elbow. J Orthop Res 1987;5(3): 372–7.
18. Sojbjerg JO, Ovesen J, Nielsen S. Experimental elbow instability after transection of the medial collateral ligament. Clin Orthop Relat Res 1987;218:186–90.
19. Morrey BF, An KN. Articular and ligamentous contributions to the stability of the elbow joint. Am J Sports Med 1983;11(5):315–9.
20. Schwab GH, Bennett JB, Woods GW, et al. Biomechanics of elbow instability: the role of the medial collateral ligament. Clin Orthop Relat Res 1980;146:42–52.
21. Callaway GH, Field LD, Deng XH, et al. Biomechanical evaluation of the medial collateral ligament of the elbow. J Bone Joint Surg Am 1997;79(8):1223–31.
22. Morrey BF, Tanaka S, An KN. Valgus stability of the elbow. A definition of primary and secondary constraints. Clin Orthop Relat Res 1991;265:187–95.
23. Ahmad CS, Park MC, ElAttrache NS. Elbow medial ulnar collateral ligament insufficiency alters posteromedial olecranon contact. Am J Sports Med 2004; 32(7):1607–12.
24. Andrews JR, Timmerman LA. Outcome of elbow surgery in professional baseball players. Am J Sports Med 1995;23(4):407–13.
25. Kamineni S, Hirahara H, Pomianowski S, et al. Partial posteromedial olecranon resection: a kinematic study. J Bone Joint Surg Am 2003;85(6):1005–11.
26. Lee YS, Alcid JG, McGarry MH, et al. Effect of olecranon resection on joint stability and strain of the medial ulnar collateral ligament. Orthopedics 2008; 31(7):648.
27. Kamineni S, ElAttrache NS, O'Driscoll SW, et al. Medial collateral ligament strain with partial posteromedial olecranon resection. A biomechanical study. J Bone Joint Surg Am 2004;86(11):2424–30.

28. Andrews JR, Heggland EJ, Fleisig GS, et al. Relationship of ulnar collateral ligament strain to amount of medial olecranon osteotomy. Am J Sports Med 2001; 29(6):716–21.

29. Levin JS, Zheng N, Dugas J, et al. Posterior olecranon resection and ulnar collateral ligament strain. J Shoulder Elbow Surg 2004;13(1):66–71.

30. Davidson PA, Pink M, Perry J, et al. Functional anatomy of the flexor pronator muscle group in relation to the medial collateral ligament of the elbow. Am J Sports Med 1995;23(2):245–50.

31. Park MC, Ahmad CS. Dynamic contributions of the flexor-pronator mass to elbow valgus stability. J Bone Joint Surg Am 2004;86(10):2268–74.

32. Udall JH, Fitzpatrick MJ, McGarry MH, et al. Effects of flexor-pronator muscle loading on valgus stability of the elbow with an intact, stretched, and resected medial ulnar collateral ligament. J Shoulder Elbow Surg 2009;18(5):773–8.

33. Lin F, Kohli N, Perlmutter S, et al. Muscle contribution to elbow joint valgus stability. J Shoulder Elbow Surg 2007;16(6):795–802.

34. Seiber K, Gupta R, McGarry MH, et al. The role of the elbow musculature, forearm rotation, and elbow flexion in elbow stability: an in vitro study. J Shoulder Elbow Surg 2009;18(2):260–8.

35. Kibler WB, Sciascia A. Kinetic chain contributions to elbow function and dysfunction in sports. Clin Sports Med 2004;23(4):545–52, viii.

36. Loftice J, Fleisig GS, Zheng N, et al. Biomechanics of the elbow in sports. Clin Sports Med 2004;23(4):519–30, vii–viii.

37. Elliott B, Fleisig G, Nicholls R, et al. Technique effects on upper limb loading in the tennis serve. J Sci Med Sport 2003;6(1):76–87.

38. Fleisig GS, Andrews JR, Dillman CJ, et al. Kinetics of baseball pitching with implications about injury mechanisms. Am J Sports Med 1995;23(2):233–9.

39. Ahmad CS, Lee TQ, ElAttrache NS. Biomechanical evaluation of a new ulnar collateral ligament reconstruction technique with interference screw fixation. Am J Sports Med 2003;31(3):332–7.

40. Bushnell BD, Anz AW, Noonan TJ, et al. Association of maximum pitch velocity and elbow injury in professional baseball pitchers. Am J Sports Med 2010;38(4): 728–32.

41. Aguinaldo AL, Chambers H. Correlation of throwing mechanics with elbow valgus load in adult baseball pitchers. Am J Sports Med 2009;37(10):2043–8.

42. Werner SL, Murray TA, Hawkins RJ, et al. Relationship between throwing mechanics and elbow valgus in professional baseball pitchers. J Shoulder Elbow Surg 2002;11(2):151–5.

43. Lyman S, Fleisig GS, Andrews JR, et al. Effect of pitch type, pitch count, and pitching mechanics on risk of elbow and shoulder pain in youth baseball pitchers. Am J Sports Med 2002;30(4):463–8.

44. Petty DH, Andrews JR, Fleisig GS, et al. Ulnar collateral ligament reconstruction in high school baseball players: clinical results and injury risk factors. Am J Sports Med 2004;32(5):1158–64.

45. Olsen SJ 2nd, Fleisig GS, Dun S, et al. Risk factors for shoulder and elbow injuries in adolescent baseball pitchers. Am J Sports Med 2006;34(6):905–12.

46. Dun S, Loftice J, Fleisig GS, et al. A biomechanical comparison of youth baseball pitches: is the curveball potentially harmful? Am J Sports Med 2008;36(4): 686–92.

47. Fleisig GS, Kingsley DS, Loftice JW, et al. Kinetic comparison among the fastball, curveball, change-up, and slider in collegiate baseball pitchers. Am J Sports Med 2006;34(3):423–30.

48. Ciccotti MC, Schwartz MA, Ciccotti MG. Diagnosis and treatment of medial epicondylitis of the elbow. Clin Sports Med 2004;23(4):693–705, xi.
49. Conway JE, Jobe FW, Glousman RE, et al. Medial instability of the elbow in throwing athletes. Treatment by repair or reconstruction of the ulnar collateral ligament. J Bone Joint Surg Am 1992;74(1):67–83.
50. Osbahr DC, Swaminathan SS, Allen AA, et al. Combined flexor-pronator mass and ulnar collateral ligament injuries in the elbows of older baseball players. Am J Sports Med 2010;38(4):733–9.
51. Osborne GV. The surgical treatment of tardy ulnar neuritis. J Bone Joint Surg Am 1957;39:782.
52. Apfelberg DB, Larson SJ. Dynamic anatomy of the ulnar nerve at the elbow. Plast Reconstr Surg 1973;51(1):79–81.
53. Aoki M, Kanaya K, Aiki H, et al. Cubital tunnel syndrome in adolescent baseball players: a report of six cases with 3- to 5-year follow-up. Arthroscopy 2005; 21(6):758.
54. Aoki M, Takasaki H, Muraki T, et al. Strain on the ulnar nerve at the elbow and wrist during throwing motion. J Bone Joint Surg Am 2005;87(11):2508–14.
55. Chen FS, Rokito AS, Jobe FW. Medial elbow problems in the overhead-throwing athlete. J Am Acad Orthop Surg 2001;9(2):99–113.
56. Ciccotti MG, Jobe FW. Medial collateral ligament instability and ulnar neuritis in the athlete's elbow. Instr Course Lect 1999;48:383–91.
57. Grana W. Medial epicondylitis and cubital tunnel syndrome in the throwing athlete. Clin Sports Med 2001;20(3):541–8.
58. Bauer M, Jonsson K, Josefsson PO, et al. Osteochondritis dissecans of the elbow. A long-term follow-up study. Clin Orthop Relat Res 1992;284: 156–60.
59. Takahara M, Shundo M, Kondo M, et al. Early detection of osteochondritis dissecans of the capitellum in young baseball players. Report of three cases. J Bone Joint Surg Am 1998;80(6):892–7.
60. Wilson FD, Andrews JR, Blackburn TA, et al. Valgus extension overload in the pitching elbow. Am J Sports Med 1983;11(2):83–8.
61. Werner SL, Fleisig GS, Dillman CJ, et al. Biomechanics of the elbow during baseball pitching. J Orthop Sports Phys Ther 1993;17(6):274–8.
62. Eygendaal D, Safran MR. Postero-medial elbow problems in the adult athlete. Br J Sports Med 2006;40(5):430–4 [discussion: 434].
63. Jones HH, Priest JD, Hayes WC, et al. Humeral hypertrophy in response to exercise. J Bone Joint Surg Am 1977;59(2):204–8.
64. Krahl H, Michaelis U, Pieper HG, et al. Stimulation of bone growth through sports. A radiologic investigation of the upper extremities in professional tennis players. Am J Sports Med 1994;22(6):751–7.
65. Chen FS, Diaz VA, Loebenberg M, et al. Shoulder and elbow injuries in the skeletally immature athlete. J Am Acad Orthop Surg 2005;13(3):172–85.
66. Rudzki JR, Paletta GA Jr. Juvenile and adolescent elbow injuries in sports. Clin Sports Med 2004;23(4):581–608, ix.
67. Han KJ, Kim YK, Lim SK, et al. The effect of physical characteristics and field position on the shoulder and elbow injuries of 490 baseball players: confirmation of diagnosis by magnetic resonance imaging. Clin J Sport Med 2009;19(4): 271–6.
68. Mihata T, Safran MR, McGarry MH, et al. Elbow valgus laxity may result in an overestimation of apparent shoulder external rotation during physical examination. Am J Sports Med 2008;36(5):978–82.

69. Thompson WH, Jobe FW, Yocum LA, et al. Ulnar collateral ligament reconstruction in athletes: muscle-splitting approach without transposition of the ulnar nerve. J Shoulder Elbow Surg 2001;10(2):152–7.

70. Timmerman LA, Schwartz ML, Andrews JR. Preoperative evaluation of the ulnar collateral ligament by magnetic resonance imaging and computed tomography arthrography. Evaluation in 25 baseball players with surgical confirmation. Am J Sports Med 1994;22(1):26–31 [discussion: 32].

71. Bennett GE. Shoulder and elbow lesions distinctive of baseball players. Ann Surg 1947;126(1):107–10.

72. King J, Brelsford HJ, Tullos HS. Analysis of the pitching arm of the professional baseball pitcher. Clin Orthop Relat Res 1969;67:116–23.

73. Dines JS, Frank JB, Akerman M, et al. Glenohumeral internal rotation deficits in baseball players with ulnar collateral ligament insufficiency. Am J Sports Med 2009;37(3):566–70.

74. Troha F, Baibak GJ, Kelleher JC. Frequency of the palmaris longus tendon in North American Caucasians. Ann Plast Surg 1990;25(6):477–8.

75. Azar FM, Andrews JR, Wilk KE, et al. Operative treatment of ulnar collateral ligament injuries of the elbow in athletes. Am J Sports Med 2000;28(1):16–23.

76. Safran MR, McGarry MH, Shin S, et al. Effects of elbow flexion and forearm rotation on valgus laxity of the elbow. J Bone Joint Surg Am 2005;87(9):2065–74.

77. O'Driscoll SW, Lawton RL, Smith AM. The "moving valgus stress test" for medial collateral ligament tears of the elbow. Am J Sports Med 2005;33(2):231–9.

78. Mulligan SA, Schwartz ML, Broussard MF, et al. Heterotopic calcification and tears of the ulnar collateral ligament: radiographic and MR imaging findings. AJR Am J Roentgenol 2000;175(4):1099–102.

79. Ellenbecker TS, Mattalino AJ, Elam EA, et al. Medial elbow joint laxity in professional baseball pitchers. A bilateral comparison using stress radiography. Am J Sports Med 1998;26(3):420–4.

80. Safran MR, Greene H, Lee TQ. Comparison of elbow valgus laxity using radiographic and non-radiographic objective measurement. 73rd Annual Meeting of the American Academy of Orthopaedic Surgeons. Chicago (IL), March 22, 2006.

81. Field LD, Altchek DW. Evaluation of the arthroscopic valgus instability test of the elbow. Am J Sports Med 1996;24(2):177–81.

82. Lee GA, Katz SD, Lazarus MD. Elbow valgus stress radiography in an uninjured population. Am J Sports Med 1998;26(3):425–7.

83. Rijke AM, Goitz HT, McCue FC, et al. Stress radiography of the medial elbow ligaments. Radiology 1994;191(1):213–6.

84. Timmerman LA, Andrews JR. Undersurface tear of the ulnar collateral ligament in baseball players. A newly recognized lesion. Am J Sports Med 1994;22(1):33–6.

85. Mirowitz SA, London SL. Ulnar collateral ligament injury in baseball pitchers: MR imaging evaluation. Radiology 1992;185(2):573–6.

86. Tuite MJ, Kijowski R. Sports-related injuries of the elbow: an approach to MRI interpretation. Clin Sports Med 2006;25(3):387–408, v.

87. Kijowski R, Tuite M, Sanford M. Magnetic resonance imaging of the elbow. Part II: abnormalities of the ligaments, tendons, and nerves. Skeletal Radiol 2005;34(1):1–18.

88. Jacobson JA, Propeck T, Jamadar DA, et al. US of the anterior bundle of the ulnar collateral ligament: findings in five cadaver elbows with MR arthrographic and anatomic comparison–initial observations. Radiology 2003;227(2):561–6.

89. Nofsinger C, Konin JG. Diagnostic ultrasound in sports medicine: current concepts and advances. Sports Med Arthrosc 2009;17(1):25–30.
90. Nazarian LN, McShane JM, Ciccotti MG, et al. Dynamic US of the anterior band of the ulnar collateral ligament of the elbow in asymptomatic major league baseball pitchers. Radiology 2003;227(1):149–54.
91. Miller TT, Adler RS, Friedman L. Sonography of injury of the ulnar collateral ligament of the elbow-initial experience. Skeletal Radiol 2004;33(7):386–91.
92. Ciccotti MG. Dynamic ultrasound of UCL. Presented at the Herodicus Society annual meeting, April 24, 2008.
93. De Smet AA, Winter TC, Best TM, et al. Dynamic sonography with valgus stress to assess elbow ulnar collateral ligament injury in baseball pitchers. Skeletal Radiol 2002;31(11):671–6.
94. Sasaki J, Takahara M, Ogino T, et al. Ultrasonographic assessment of the ulnar collateral ligament and medial elbow laxity in college baseball players. J Bone Joint Surg Am 2002;84(4):525–31.
95. Rettig AC, Sherrill C, Snead DS, et al. Nonoperative treatment of ulnar collateral ligament injuries in throwing athletes. Am J Sports Med 2001;29(1):15–7.
96. Barnes DA, Tullos HS. An analysis of 100 symptomatic baseball players. Am J Sports Med 1978;6(2):62–7.
97. Richard MJ, Aldridge JM 3rd, Wiesler ER, et al. Traumatic valgus instability of the elbow: pathoanatomy and results of direct repair. Surgical technique. J Bone Joint Surg Am 2009;91(Suppl 2):191–9.
98. Richard MJ, Aldridge JM 3rd, Wiesler ER, et al. Traumatic valgus instability of the elbow: pathoanatomy and results of direct repair. J Bone Joint Surg Am 2008;90(11):2416–22.
99. Savoie FH 3rd, Trenhaile SW, Roberts J, et al. Primary repair of ulnar collateral ligament injuries of the elbow in young athletes: a case series of injuries to the proximal and distal ends of the ligament. Am J Sports Med 2008;36(6):1066–72.
100. Gibson BW, Webner D, Huffman GR, et al. Ulnar collateral ligament reconstruction in major league baseball pitchers. Am J Sports Med 2007;35(4):575–81.
101. Jobe FW, Stark H, Lombardo SJ. Reconstruction of the ulnar collateral ligament in athletes. J Bone Joint Surg Am 1986;68(8):1158–63.
102. Purcell DB, Matava MJ, Wright RW. Ulnar collateral ligament reconstruction: a systematic review. Clin Orthop Relat Res 2007;455:72–7.
103. Meyers A, Palmer B, Baratz ME. Ulnar collateral ligament reconstruction. Hand Clin 2008;24(1):53–67.
104. Smith GR, Altchek DW, Pagnani MJ, et al. A muscle-splitting approach to the ulnar collateral ligament of the elbow. Neuroanatomy and operative technique. Am J Sports Med 1996;24(5):575–80.
105. Rohrbough JT, Altchek DW, Hyman J, et al. Medial collateral ligament reconstruction of the elbow using the docking technique. Am J Sports Med 2002;30(4):541–8.
106. Ciccotti MG, Siegler S, Kuri JA 2nd, et al. Comparison of the biomechanical profile of the intact ulnar collateral ligament with the modified Jobe and the Docking reconstructed elbow: an in vitro study. Am J Sports Med 2009;37(5):974–81.
107. Koh JL, Schafer MF, Keuter G, et al. Ulnar collateral ligament reconstruction in elite throwing athletes. Arthroscopy 2006;22(11):1187–91.
108. Paletta GA Jr, Wright RW. The modified docking procedure for elbow ulnar collateral ligament reconstruction: 2-year follow-up in elite throwers. Am J Sports Med 2006;34(10):1594–8.

109. Paletta GA Jr, Klepps SJ, Difelice GS, et al. Biomechanical evaluation of 2 techniques for ulnar collateral ligament reconstruction of the elbow. Am J Sports Med 2006;34(10):1599–603.

110. Hurbanek JG, Anderson K, Crabtree S, et al. Biomechanical comparison of the docking technique with and without humeral bioabsorbable interference screw fixation. Am J Sports Med 2009;37(3):526–33.

111. Large TM, Coley ER, Peindl RD, et al. A biomechanical comparison of 2 ulnar collateral ligament reconstruction techniques. Arthroscopy 2007; 23(2):141–50.

112. McAdams TR, Lee AT, Centeno J, et al. Two ulnar collateral ligament reconstruction methods: the docking technique versus bioabsorbable interference screw fixation–a biomechanical evaluation with cyclic loading. J Shoulder Elbow Surg 2007;16(2):224–8.

113. Conway JE. The DANE TJ procedure for elbow medial ulnar collateral ligament insufficiency. Tech Shoulder Elbow Surg 2006;7(1):36–43.

114. Dines JS, ElAttrache NS, Conway JE, et al. Clinical outcomes of the DANE TJ technique to treat ulnar collateral ligament insufficiency of the elbow. Am J Sports Med 2007;35(12):2039–44.

115. Armstrong AD, Dunning CE, Ferreira LM, et al. A biomechanical comparison of four reconstruction techniques for the medial collateral ligament-deficient elbow. J Shoulder Elbow Surg 2005;14(2):207–15.

116. Ruland RT, Hogan CJ, Randall CJ, et al. Biomechanical comparison of ulnar collateral ligament reconstruction techniques. Am J Sports Med 2008;36(8). 1565–70.

117. Shah RP, Lindsey DP, Sungar GW, et al. An analysis of four ulnar collateral ligament reconstruction procedures with cyclic valgus loading. J Shoulder Elbow Surg 2009;18(1):58–63.

118. Lee GH, Limpisvasti O, Park MC, et al. Revision ulnar collateral ligament reconstruction using a suspension button fixation technique. Am J Sports Med 2010; 38(3):575–80.

119. Hechtman KS, Tjin-A-Tsoi EW, Zvijac JE, et al. Biomechanics of a less invasive procedure for reconstruction of the ulnar collateral ligament of the elbow. Am J Sports Med 1998;26(5):620–4.

120. Bernas GA, Ruberte Thiele RA, Kinnaman KA, et al. Defining safe rehabilitation for ulnar collateral ligament reconstruction of the elbow: a biomechanical study. Am J Sports Med 2009;37(12):2392–400.

121. Domb BG, Davis JT, Alberta FG, et al. Clinical follow-up of professional baseball players undergoing ulnar collateral ligament reconstruction using the new Kerlan-Jobe Orthopaedic Clinic Overhead Athlete Shoulder and Elbow Score (KJOC Score). Am J Sports Med 2010;38(8):1558–63.

122. Vitale MA, Ahmad CS. The outcome of elbow ulnar collateral ligament reconstruction in overhead athletes: a systematic review. Am J Sports Med 2008; 36(6):1193–205.

123. Andrews JR. Complications of ulnar collateral ligament reconstruction. Presented at the International Society of Arthroscopy, Knee Surgery and Orthopedic Sports Medicine (ISAKOS). Florence (Italy), May 30, 2007.

124. Dines JS, Yocum LA, Frank JB, et al. Revision surgery for failed elbow medial collateral ligament reconstruction. Am J Sports Med 2008;36(6):1061–5.

125. Argo D, Trenhaile SW, Savoie FH 3rd, et al. Operative treatment of ulnar collateral ligament insufficiency of the elbow in female athletes. Am J Sports Med 2006;34(3):431–7.

126. Dodson CC, Nho SJ, Williams RJ 3rd, et al. Elbow arthroscopy. J Am Acad Orthop Surg 2008;16(10):574–85.

127. Steinmann SP. Elbow arthroscopy: where are we now? Arthroscopy 2007;23(11): 1231–6.

128. O'Driscoll SW, Morrey BF. Arthroscopy of the elbow. Diagnostic and therapeutic benefits and hazards. J Bone Joint Surg Am 1992;74(1):84–94.

Valgus Extension Overload: Diagnosis and Treatment

Jeffrey R. Dugas, MD

KEYWORDS

• Valgus extension overload • Posterior impingement
• Olecranon stress fracture • Thrower's elbow • Stress fracture
• Olecranon apophyseal nonunion

Injuries to the thrower's elbow have become commonplace in the adult, adolescent, and even youth sports arenas. In fact, there has been a nearly 10-fold increase in the number of surgical reconstructions of the ulnar collateral ligament in throwing athletes in the last 10 years. Predictable factors leading to the increase in injury rates have been published repeatedly, but the available data do not support a decrease in the injury rates at this time. Among throwing athletes, the shoulder and the elbow are, by far, the most often injured anatomic areas of the body. This prevalence is caused by the tremendous forces generated in these body areas in the course of the throwing motion. To understand the injury patterns and their treatment options, as well as the possible prevention of the injuries, we must understand the anatomy of the anatomic areas of interest, along with the biomechanics and pathomechanics that lead to the common injuries.

Valgus extension overload (VEO) is a syndrome of symptoms and physical findings that are commonly seen in the throwing or overhead athlete. In a review of the results of elbow surgery in 72 professional baseball players, the most common pathology seen was olecranon osteophytes, which was found in 65% of the cases.[1] In 2000, Reddy and colleagues[2] published a series of nearly 200 elbow arthroscopies in which more than 50% had posterior impingement. Some nonthrowers who frequently suffer from VEO are swimmers, volleyball players, gymnasts, racquet-sport athletes, and golfers. VEO is a condition that results from impingement of the posteromedial tip of the olecranon process on the medial wall of the olecranon fossa. This part of the elbow articulation is normally conforming, making abnormal tracking or impingement unlikely. However, in the overhead athlete or throwing athlete, some increase in medial elbow laxity may predispose the athlete to micromotion of the olecranon tip within the fossa as the elbow is forcibly extended. King and colleagues[3] suggested that with excessive valgus force, ligamentous laxity on the medial aspect of the elbow accentuates the

American Sports Medicine Institute, 2660 10th Avenue South, Suite 505, Birmingham, AL 35205, USA
E-mail address: Kelsey.mclemore@andrewscenters.com

Clin Sports Med 29 (2010) 645–654
doi:10.1016/j.csm.2010.07.001
0278-5919/10/$ – see front matter © 2010 Elsevier Inc. All rights reserved.

impingement of the posteromedial olecranon within the olecranon fossa. This posteromedial impingement, over a course of time, leads to osteophyte formation on the posteromedial tip of the olecranon as the body attempts to create more stability. With continued throwing or overhead delivery, the impingement and the symptoms of the condition worsen. In the pages to follow, the author reviews the critical anatomy and pathology of VEO, the process of diagnosis, and both conservative and surgical management in the athlete. The author also reviews some of the factors that lead to an increase in injury risk, and some preventative measures that can help an athlete to avoid VEO and other conditions common to the overhead athlete.

VEO HISTORY AND PATHOLOGY

Osteophytes do not occur rapidly, but rather require a significant time to form, likely in the months-to-years timeline rather than the days-to-weeks timeline. For this reason, it is important to understand the condition of the elbow leading up to the onset of symptoms and the pathomechanics that lead to the initial insult.

The ulnar collateral ligament of the elbow (UCL), commonly called the Tommy John ligament after the baseball pitcher who first underwent successful UCL reconstruction, is the main ligamentous stabilizer to the medial or inside part of the elbow. With each overhead throw, the elbow experiences an average of 64 Nm of valgus stress, of which approximately 50% is taken up by the UCL.[4] The rapid elbow extension that occurs with throwing is one of the fastest recorded human motions, the endpoint of which occurs as the tip of the olecranon is forced into its counterpart, the olecranon fossa. With any increased laxity or injury to the UCL, there is a compensatory increase in compression on the medial aspect of the olecranon-olecranon fossa articulation as the elbow is forcibly extended. It is not necessary for the UCL to rupture completely for such an increase to occur. Any injury that creates even the smallest increase in medial laxity may eventually lead to VEO. Such conditions may occur and exist as early as the youngest ages of throwing, but may not become evident as VEO until much later. If a youth thrower were to experience a minimal medial epicondyle injury, a slight distal migration of the epicondyle (and its UCL origin) could lead to increased valgus laxity and subsequent increase in pressure posteromedially with terminal extension. If a thrower were to experience a ligament strain, it is possible for such an injury to lead to some increase in laxity of the ligament, which over time could lead to VEO.

Aguinaldo and Chambers[5] reported in 2009 on several mechanical factors in the throwing motion that predispose the elbow to high valgus load. These factors include late trunk rotation, reduced shoulder external rotation, and increased elbow flexion. Sidearm pitchers were found to be more susceptible than overhand pitchers. Many throwers and overhead athletes never get to the point of having a clinical problem with VEO because they discontinue throwing in high volumes as the result of increasing age and decreasing opportunity to play competitive overhead sports beyond adolescence and early adulthood. In higher-level athletes, and those who continue to enjoy overhead sports into adulthood, the likelihood of developing symptomatic VEO is increased. Recurrent UCL injuries, such as strains or minimal tears, can lead to increased laxity and subsequent increase in contact pressure in the posteromedial aspect of the elbow in extension.

DIAGNOSIS

As is true with many of the pathologic conditions commonly seen in throwing athletes, VEO can typically be diagnosed with a thorough history and physical examination, and confirmed with simple radiographic tests or, if necessary, more sophisticated tests like MRI. The first order of business when addressing any thrower with an injury is to obtain an adequate history of the symptoms related to the athlete. Among the more important questions to ask a thrower is when in the course of the throwing motion the symptoms occur. This question will help focus the examination and thought process. If the athlete experiences pain medially at the onset of arm acceleration, there should be concern about the UCL. If the athlete experiences posterior pain at ball release when the elbow nears terminal extension, VEO is more likely to be the cause. Not all posterior pain at ball release is caused by VEO, but the *typical* history of VEO is pain at ball release. Another question that may help delineate the cause of symptoms is whether any activity other than throwing causes symptoms. Posteromedial pain with resisted arm extension may be more likely with distal triceps tendonitis rather than VEO.

On physical examination, the examiner should proceed through a normal elbow examination (including inspection, range of motion, strength testing, stability testing, and neurovascular examination), and then proceed to specific testing for VEO. Keep in mind that valgus stress testing of the elbow in 20° of elbow flexion is designed to simulate the stress on the UCL. The specific test for VEO is accomplished by repeatedly placing a valgus stress on the elbow at 20° to 30° of flexion while forcing the elbow into terminal extension (**Fig. 1**A, B). It is important for the examiner to know

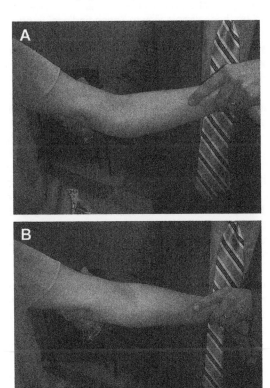

Fig. 1. Clinical photographs of the physical examination of the elbow demonstrating the test for VEO. With this test, the examiner attempts to recreate the symptoms by grasping the wrist with the elbow in 20° to 30° of flexion (*A*), and forcibly extending the elbow while applying a valgus stress (*B*).

that it is common for a thrower to have some loss of elbow extension in the dominant throwing elbow, and this finding should not affect the examiner's process of examination. Also, the examiner should ask the athlete if pain with the VEO test causes a reproduction of the pain or symptoms they experience during throwing, and if those symptoms occur at the posteromedial tip of the olecranon process, which can be easily palpated by the examiner. All patients suspected of having an injury to the UCL should be evaluated for VEO. The presence or absence of posteromedial pain in forced extension should be noted in the physical examination of each thrower.

Careful examination of the other susceptible structures on the medial side of the elbow should be performed by the examiner at this time. Specifically, palpation of the ulnar nerve, the UCL, the distal medial triceps, and the flexor-pronator group should be conducted to ensure that these structures are not involved in the process. The examiner should ensure that the ulnar nerve is stable within the cubital tunnel throughout the range of motion, and that no ulnar nerve-distribution symptoms are present.

Plain radiographs of the elbow should be taken, including the standard anteroposterior (AP), lateral, and axial views (**Fig. 2**). In the author's facility, it is preferred to obtain 2 oblique views as well as the standard 3 views previously noted. If necessary, views of the contralateral uninvolved elbow may be done for comparison purposes. As seen in **Fig. 3**, the presence of a posteromedial olecranon osteophyte or loose body should be visualized on these simple views. These findings, in addition to the history and physical examination, help to confirm the diagnosis of VEO. As previously noted, VEO is a syndrome of symptoms, not a radiographic condition. The absence of osteophytes or loose bodies does *not* eliminate VEO as a cause of the athletes' symptoms, because the condition of posteromedial impingement predates the formation of osteophytes.

Sophisticated tests, such as MRI, may be indicated if the diagnosis is in question or to confirm the suspicion of the clinician based upon history, physical examination, and radiographs. MRI will likely demonstrate the condition of the UCL, which may be important in some throwers who have a history of UCL injury, which may have lead to the presence of VEO. MRI will also typically demonstrate the presence or absence of loose bodies within the elbow joint and the presence or absence of osteophytes on the posteromedial tip of the olecranon process. In cases where the condition of the UCL is uncertain, MRI should be used to determine if there is a significant injury. If the athlete would benefit from UCL reconstruction, excision of the posteromedial tip of the olecranon can be performed during the UCL reconstruction. This information should obviously be determined before any surgical intervention.

The ulnar nerve can also be the source of posteromedial pain within the cubital tunnel. Instability of the ulnar nerve can typically be demonstrated on physical examination, and in many cases it can be visualized as patients flex their elbow beyond 90°. Pain with ulnar nerve palpation is not always accompanied by ulnar nerve-distribution sensory symptoms. A careful examination of the nerve as opposed to the posteromedial tip of the olecranon should allow the examiner to distinguish between these 2 clinical entities.

Forced extension from throwing can also lead to proximal olecranon stress fractures in throwing athletes. These injuries can be the result of excessive tensile stress from the triceps tendon, repetitive microtrauma, and posterior impingement of the olecranon against the olecranon fossa.[6] In these cases, symptoms may occur during or *after* throwing, and may be more insidious in onset than other elbow pathology. Pain to palpation is typically more distal and lateral on the proximal shaft of the olecranon rather than posteromedial as is seen in VEO. Forced extension may also elicit

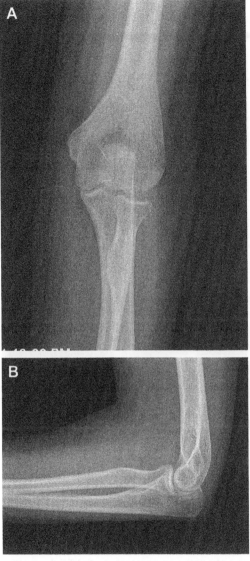

Fig. 2. Plain radiographs of a normal elbow, including a standard AP view (*A*) and a standard lateral view (*B*).

pain with these types of injuries, which may make it difficult to distinguish from VEO. If plain radiographs are suggestive of an olecranon stress fracture, a CT scan, MRI, or bone scan may be used to confirm the findings (**Fig. 4**).

TREATMENT

Athletes who present with symptoms consistent with isolated VEO (no UCL issues) should be managed with active rest. Active rest includes rest from throwing and other inciting activities, along with specific exercises to increase rotator cuff strength, flexor-pronator strength, and improved mechanics. Nonsteroidal antiinflammatory medications

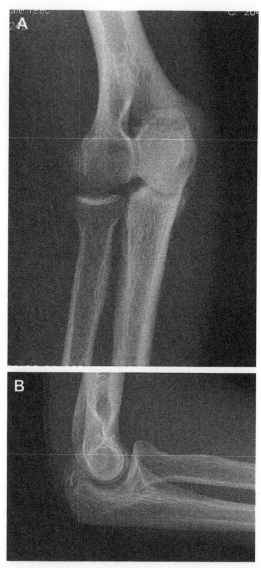

Fig. 3. Plain radiographs of a patient with symptomatic VEO demonstrating a typical poster-omedial olecranon osteophyte on both the AP view (*A*) and the lateral view (*B*).

may also be used for a specified period of time. In first-time throwers with VEO, we will typically remove them from throwing for 10 to 14 days, followed by a gradual return to throwing through an interval throwing program. In those who have had multiple episodes of symptoms, a more prolonged period of rest (4–6 weeks) may be indicated, followed by a more gradual interval throwing program. We have not found corticosteroid injection to be useful in the management of these conditions, although it is unlikely that any harm is done by administering a single intraarticular dose of soluble corticosteroid.

Athletes with olecranon stress fractures or unfused olecranon apophyses are treated in a similar manner as previously described. First, the athlete should discontinue throwing and begin a course of active rest, avoiding any exercise that causes

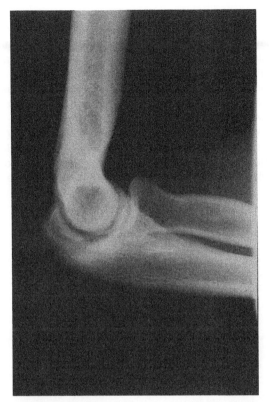

Fig. 4. Typical lateral radiograph of a proximal olecranon stress fracture.

discomfort. After several weeks, a plyometric program may be initiated, followed by an interval throwing program and gradual return to competition.

If conservative management is not effective in relieving the symptoms, surgical management may be considered. Typical surgical management consists of routine elbow arthroscopy with thorough inspection of all aspects of the elbow joint. Unless we have a need to do so, we typically will *not* make an anteromedial portal. When working posteriorly, we make a posterolateral portal and place the arthroscope in this portal to view the posterior compartment of the elbow. From this position, a posteromedial portal is established under spinal needle localization. This portal is typically made as close to the medial border of the distal triceps as possible to avoid inadvertent injury to the nearby ulnar nerve. Once the position of the portal is established with a needle, a 5 to 7 mm incision is made longitudinally in the skin and blunt dissection is carried down to the posterior joint capsule, again to avoid injury to the nearby ulnar nerve. A blunt trocar is used to gain access to the posterior elbow and, once completely established, instruments to remove loose bodies or osteophytes can be used through this portal. If necessary, the arthroscope can be switched to the posteromedial portal and instruments can be used through the posterolateral portal. At the author's institution, making a transtriceps portal in throwing athletes is avoided because this may be a source of pain as the arm is forcefully extended in the act of throwing. Also, this portal tends to cause increased postoperative pain and can limit early range of motion, particularly in elbow flexion.

We typically use an arthroscopic shaver or burr to remove the posteromedial tip of the olecranon. We may also use a 4 mm osteotome to remove some or all of the abnormal bone. Several studies have shown that it is safe to remove the tip of the olecranon without placing increased stress on the UCL. Several clinical and basic science studies have been published regarding the amount of bone to be resected and the effect on the remaining tissues.[7,8] In a study by Levin and colleagues,[7] it was demonstrated that up to 8 mm of olecranon may be resected safely without an increase in strain on the UCL with valgus stress applied.

Fig. 5 demonstrates the typical arthroscopic view of the impinging posterior osteophyte before and after resection. Careful inspection of the articular surface of the trochlea is performed through a range of motion to ensure that there are no full-thickness areas of cartilage loss, which is not infrequently seen in these cases. If there is full-thickness loss, it is typically in the posteromedial trochlea and is treated with microfracture at the time of osteophyte removal.

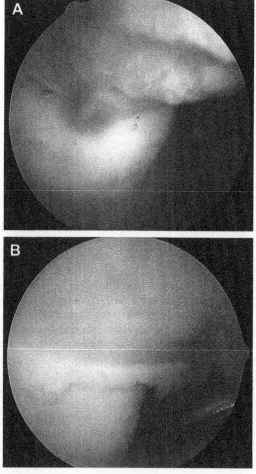

Fig. 5. Plain radiographs obtained after arthroscopic resection of the symptomatic osteophyte in a patient with VEO.

Once the resection is completed and no further intraarticular pathology remains, the arthroscopic instruments are removed and the portals are closed with simple sutures. At the author's institution, patients are typically placed in a posterior splint for 3 to 5 days to allow the portals to begin to heal before removing the splint and starting gentle range-of-motion exercises. At the completion of the procedure, a plain lateral radiograph is obtained to ensure that the entire osteophyte has been removed and that no further bony fragments remain in the elbow. This radiograph is taken in the operating room, before removing drapes and awakening patients from anesthesia. In this way, a proper amount of olecranon resection is ensured.

In cases of olecranon stress fracture or unfused olecranon apophysis, if rest and conservative management fail to return the athlete to competition, surgical intervention should be considered. The standard surgical technique for olecranon stress fractures is a single, large, cannulated, partially threaded screw inserted antegrade through the distal triceps via a small (1 cm) longitudinal incision. Fluoroscopic guidance is used to ensure that the threads of the screw are all distal to the stress fracture and that the entire screw is intramedullary, which ensures adequate compression across the area of interest.

For the first 2 weeks, the recovery from arthroscopic resection is centered on edema control and regaining range of motion. By the 2-week point, the portals have typically healed and the sutures have been removed. Range of motion will typically be back to normal by the 3- to 4-week point. At the 4- to 6-week point, we typically begin some plyometric exercises designed to gently stress the tissues around the elbow joint, specifically the UCL. This plyometric program continues for 4 to 6 weeks, at which time the athlete is allowed to begin the interval throwing program. Completion of the interval throwing program may take anywhere from several weeks to several months depending on the level of competition and the ability of the individual athlete. Typically, an athlete undergoing uncomplicated arthroscopic resection will return to competition anywhere between 3 and 6 months postoperatively, which is in stark contrast to the average of 12 months for return to competition from the typical UCL reconstruction.

For olecranon stress fractures, bony union typically takes at least 8 weeks, but may be delayed. Once healed completely, gradual stress and return to activity is initiated. In some recalcitrant cases, a bone stimulator may be helpful in obtaining complete bony union. Once the plyometric program is complete (usually around 3 months after surgery), the interval throwing program is initiated, followed by return to throwing. Expected return to competition following fixation of these injuries is typically 6 months.

In a large review of more than 1200 UCL reconstructions, there was a 7% incidence of previous olecranon tip excision in the reconstructed group.[9] In the same study, 23% of subjects undergoing UCL reconstruction had concomitant olecranon tip excision, and 5% of the subjects who had already undergone UCL reconstruction underwent subsequent olecranon tip excision at a later time. What is unclear from these data is whether the early insults to the UCL led to symptomatic VEO, or if the treatment of VEO led to the UCL injury. This "which came first, the chicken or the egg?" debate is unresolved at this point. However, the author believes that these conditions are in the same spectrum of injury and likely occur concurrently in many throwers. Recurrence of the symptoms or clinical findings of VEO are rare and have not been reported in any of the large series of elbow procedures in athletes. In the author's clinical experience, recurrence of posteromedial impingement is secondary to an underappreciation of the underlying medial ligamentous laxity and other predisposing pathology.

Regardless of cause, the careful management of VEO and other posterior elbow pathology should lead to successful return to competitive throwing or overhead sports.

The first published report of a group of throwing athletes was by Wilson and colleagues[10] in 1983. In their review of 5 subjects who underwent open excision of the osteophyte, all 5 were able to return for at least 1 full year of competition at maximum effectiveness. Since that time, other reports have demonstrated similar rates of return to competition. The key to success with VEO is the early recognition of the condition and the careful conservative management of the symptoms with appropriate periods of rest. If those conservative measures fail, arthroscopic surgical management is typically successful in returning the athlete to competitive sports at all levels.

REFERENCES

1. Andrews JR, Timmerman LA. Outcome of elbow surgery in professional baseball players. Am J Sports Med 1995;23:407–13.
2. Reddy AS, Kvitne RS, Yocum LA, et al. Arthroscopy of the elbow: a long-term clinical review. Arthroscopy 2000;16:588–94.
3. King JW, Brelsford HJ, Tullos HS. Analysis of the pitching arm of the professional baseball pitcher. Clin Orthop 1969;67:116–23.
4. Fleisig GS, Andrws JR, Dillman CJ, et al. Kinetics of baseball pitching with implications about injury mechanisms. Am J Sports Med 1995;23:233–9.
5. Aguinaldo AL, Chambers H. Correlation of throwing mechanics with elbow valgus load in adult baseball pitchers. Am J Sports Med 2009;37:2043–8.
6. Griggs SM, Weiss AP. Bony injuries of the wrist, forearm, and elbow. Clin Sports Med 1996;15:373–400.
7. Levin JS, Zheng N, Dugas JR, et al. Posterior olecranon resection and ulnar collateral ligament strain. J Shoulder Elbow Surg 2004;13(1):66–71.
8. Andrews JR, Heggland EJ, Fleisig GS, et al. Relationship of ulnar collateral ligament strain to amount of medial olecranon osteotomy. Am J Sports Med 2001;29:716–21.
9. Cain EL Jr, Andrews JR, Dugas JR, et al. Ulnar collateral ligament reconstruction: a review of over 1200 cases. Am J Sports Med, submitted for publication.
10. Wilson FD, Andrews JR, Blackburn TA, et al. Valgus extension overload in the pitching elbow. Am J Sports Med 1983;11:83–8.

Nerve Injuries About the Elbow

Sanaz Hariri, MD[a], Timothy R. McAdams, MD[b],*

KEYWORDS

- Athlete's elbow • Neuropathy • Cubital tunnel syndrome
- Pronator syndrome • Radial tunnel syndrome
- Posterior interosseous nerve syndrome

Athletes rely on their elbows to place their hand in space and to transfer force down the arm. Although throwing athletes are at particular risk, any athlete involved in lifting, pushing, pulling, or transferring force to a hand-held piece of equipment (eg, a racquet) is at risk for an elbow injury. High repetitive stress placed on the elbow during athletics may cause traction injuries to nerves traversing the region. Sources of compression on nerves, heightened by the strain of athletics, may also cause neuropathy. This article presents a review of the cause, pathology, work-up, and treatment options for nerve injuries about the elbow in athletes. The work-up for these disorders must include an evaluation of the entire length of the nerve being investigated, from the cervical spine to its terminal branches. During the work-up, one must also be mindful that a single nerve may be compressed at more than one level (double crush).

CUBITAL TUNNEL SYNDROME

Cubital tunnel syndrome (CuTS) is a compressive neuropathy of the ulnar nerve (comprised of C8 and T1 nerve root fibers from the medial cord of the brachial plexus) at the cubital tunnel. The superficial location and anatomy of the ulnar nerve at the elbow make CuTS the second most common entrapment neuropathy of the upper extremity (carpal tunnel syndrome being the most common). The differential diagnosis for CuTS includes sites of ulnar nerve compression more proximally (including C8 nerve root entrapment, thoracic outlet syndrome, compression of the ulnar nerve at the arcade of Struthers), medial epicondylitis, and ulnar collateral ligament (UCL) injury.

Funding support: none.
[a] Sports Medicine, Orthopaedic Surgery, Stanford University, 1169 Trinity Drive, Menlo Park, CA 94025, USA
[b] Orthopaedic Surgery, Stanford University, 450 Broadway Street, M/C 6120, Redwood City, CA 94063, USA
* Corresponding author.
E-mail address: tmcadams@stanford.edu

Proximal to the elbow, the ulnar nerve pierces through the medial intermuscular septum to move from the anterior to posterior compartment. It then passes through the arcade of Struthers about 8 cm proximal to the medial epicondyle. At the elbow, the nerve passes between the medial epicondyle and the olecranon. It then enters the cubital tunnel, formed by the UCL, the medial edge of the trochlea, and the medial epicondylar groove. The arcuate ligament (also called the cubital tunnel retinaculum) extends from the medial epicondyle to the medial aspect of the olecranon and forms the roof of the cubital tunnel, holding the ulnar nerve within the tunnel. The cubital tunnel is 4 mm wide and has transversely oriented fibers that are perpendicular to the flexor carpi ulnaris (FCU) aponeurosis, which blends with its distal margin. The arcuate ligament is lax in extension and taut in elbow flexion. It is perhaps a remnant of the anconeus epitrochlearis muscle (an anomalous muscle arising from the medial border of the olecranon and the adjacent triceps and inserting on the medial epicondyle). In some cases, the anconeus epitrochlearis muscle replaces the arcuate ligament.[1]

The nerve then passes between the 2 heads of the FCU and courses into the forearm. Its motor nerve innervations distal to the cubital tunnel include: the FCU, the medial half of the flexor digitorum profundus (FDP), most of the hand intrinsic muscles, and some of the hypothenar eminence muscles. It provides sensation to the dorsal and palmar surfaces of the fourth and fifth digits and the ulnar border of the hand.[2]

There are many potential sources of CuTS (**Box 1**, **Fig. 1**). Compression is the major mechanism of ulnar neuropathy in the cubital tunnel. Even in the normal elbow, the ulnar nerve undergoes considerable traction and compression deformation with range of motion. The tunnel has its maximum capacity in full elbow extension when the arcuate ligament is slack. In full extension, the relaxed ulnar nerve follows a tortuous course. For every 45° of elbow flexion, the arcuate ligament stretches about 5 mm, reducing the cross-sectional area of the cubital tunnel. With increasing elbow flexion, the course of the nerve becomes progressively linear, and the usually round nerve shifts anteriorly in the cubital tunnel, eventually becoming flattened against the medial epicondyle. The nerve is on maximal tension with full elbow flexion and forearm pronation.[2,3]

Anatomic extrinsic sources of compression, some varying by sport, can compound the intrinsic compression caused by the anatomy of the cubital tunnel. Pitchers may have hypertrophied flexor muscles that can compress the ulnar nerve.[2] Athletes who have hypertrophy of the medial head of the biceps and/or the origin of the pronator flexor muscles (eg, weight-lifters) are also predisposed to CuTS. Rarely, an anconeus epitrochlearis muscle may cause CuTS.[5,6]

CuTS may be caused by traction on the ulnar nerve during the throwing motion. Within 20° of extension and during flexion more than 120°, bony anatomy is the primary elbow stabilizing structure. Between 20° and 120°, the medial soft tissue is the primary constraint to valgus force during the throwing motion, particularly the anterior bundle of the UCL. The medial elbow structures, including the ulnar nerve, are subjected to forces as high as 64 N m during the throwing motion.[7] The repetitive, forceful activities of throwers (eg, pitchers) and overhead athletes (eg, tennis, volleyball) can compromise ulnar nerve function. For example, volleyball players engage in spiking and serving with their dominant arm. The motor conduction velocity of the ulnar nerve at the elbow is significantly delayed in the dominant arms of even asymptomatic volleyball players compared with their own nondominant arms and with nonathletes.[8]

The repetitive elbow flexion, extension, and valgus stress experienced by throwing athletes may damage the UCL. Stretch or tearing of the UCL leads to joint laxity, increasing nerve motility within the groove and leading to stretch, compression, and/or subluxation. Injury to the UCL can also cause inflammation, thickening, adhesions, and subsequent neuropathy. Medial traction osteophytes may deform the groove, compressing or irritating the ulnar nerve.[9] Contact athletes (eg, wrestlers, rugby, and football players) are also at risk because the superficial location of the nerve leaves it vulnerable to direct trauma.

Athletes with CuTS complain of pain along the medial aspect of the elbow during throwing and overhead activities accompanied by numbness and/or tingling in the ulnar forearm, the ulnar border of the hand, and the ring and small fingers. Later, hand weakness may develop, manifesting as clumsiness of the hand and fingers while throwing. There may be night pain caused by full elbow flexion during sleep.[2] McGowan defined 3 grades of ulnar neuritis in 1950. Grade 1 lesions are minimal, with no detectable motor weakness of the hand. Grade 2 lesions are intermediate. Grade 3 lesions are severe, with paralysis of 1 or more of the ulnar intrinsic muscles.[10] Initially, symptoms are present only during activities such as throwing. As ulnar nerve damage progresses, symptoms become more constant, occurring even at rest, and visible atrophy of the interosseous hand muscles may develop.

The examination should include a test for ulnar neuropathy and tests to exclude other pathologies should also be performed. Full bilateral upper extremity strength examinations should look for signs of other compressive neuropathies, brachial plexus injury, and cervical radiculopathy. The alignment of the upper extremity should be examined, looking for cubitus valgus, an elbow contracture, and muscular hypertrophy. Elbow range of motion and stability (particularly on valgus stress with the elbow in about 30° of flexion) should be tested. A motor examination should focus on muscles innervated by the ulnar nerve distal to the cubital tunnel: forearm flexors (the FCU and ulnar portion of FDP), the hypothenar eminence, and hand intrinsics (Table 1). The patient may not be able to adduct the little finger (Wartenberg sign). Severe intrinsic weakness manifests as a claw hand deformity (flexion of the ring and small finger proximal and distal interphalangeal [PIP and DIP] joints with extension of those metacarpal phalangeal [MCP] joints). However, throwing and overhead athletes often have hypertrophied musculature, making relative weakness difficult to discern. A hand dynamometer may be used over time to document progressive loss of strength.

A sensory examination should include the lateral forearm, the small finger, and the ulnar side of the ring finger. A 2-point discrimination test can be performed on the affected fingers and compared with the other digits. The nerve should be palpated within the cubital tunnel and then palpated with elbow flexion to detect anterior subluxation/dislocation. Provocative tests may also be performed to elicit signs of ulnar neuropathy, including the Froment sign, the elbow-flexion test, and the Tinel sign (Table 2). Certain maneuvers are used to rule out other pathologic conditions. In medial epicondylitis, there is tenderness over the flexor pronator tendon origin that increases with resisted wrist flexion and forearm pronation. UCL injury manifests as pain reproducible with valgus stress on the elbow.

Plain films of the elbow should be obtained to look for any bony anatomic sources of impingement, such as a fracture malunion or an osteophyte. If the diagnosis is unclear, electrodiagnostic testing (usually a nerve conduction study [NCS], but sometimes also an electromyogram [EMG]) should be considered to localize the lesion and determine the severity of nerve damage, although there is a significant false-negative rate.[2,11] The sensitivity of these tests may be improved if performed after throwing.[12] Ultrasonography can also be used to detect swelling of a compressed nerve and to visualize the cause of compression (eg, a ganglion or an anconeus epitrochlearis muscle).[13] A

Box 1
Causes of CuTS

1. Five classic sources of compression

   Arcade of Struthers

   Medial intermuscular septum

   Medial epicondyle

   The cubital tunnel itself with Osborne band (tendinous proximal edge of the flexor carpi ulnaris muscle)

   Deep flexor pronator aponeurosis

2. Other anatomic sources of compression/traction

   Medial head of the flexor carpi ulnaris (FCU)

   Malunion of the distal ulnar or epiphyseal injury with subsequent cubitus valgus

   Space-occupying lesions within the cubital tunnel: eg, ganglia, osteophytes, and neoplasms (eg, lipomas or neurolemmoma)

   Thickening, scarring, or calcification of the ulnar collateral ligament at the floor of the tunnel

3. Congenital anatomic factors

   Congenital hypoplasia of the trochlea

   Congenital cubitus valgus

   Anconeus epitrochlearis muscle (originates from humerus' medial epicondyle, inserts onto the ulna's olecranon process)

   Abnormal insertion of the medial head of the triceps muscle into the medial epicondyle[4]

4. External sources

   Blunt trauma/direct blow

   Elbow dislocation

   Recurrent trauma (eg, repeated elbow resting on hard surfaces)

   Fracture of the medial humeral epicondyle

5. Dynamic sources

   Subluxation of the ulnar nerve and/or triceps muscle

6. Metabolic or endocrine disease causing local swelling

   Diabetes mellitus

   Alcoholism

   Hypothyroidism

   Renal disease

   Hansen disease

   Uremia

   Amyloidosis

   Mucoppolysaccharidosis

   Acromegaly

   Pregnancy

   Pseudotumoral calcinosis

7. Systemic disease

   Rheumatoid arthritis

   Systemic erythematosus lupus (SLE)

   Scleroderma

8. Occupational/overuse factors

   Keyboard operators (elbow flexion, resting elbows on hard surface)

   Excessive driving (arm abducted, elbow flexed, forearm pronated, elbow may be resting on the window or armrest)

Data from Norkus SA, Meyers MC. Ulnar neuropathy of the elbow. Sports Med 1994;17(3): 189–99.

magnetic resonance imaging (MRI) scan can be ordered if UCL or a pathologic condition originating in the flexor-pronator tendon is suspected (**Figs. 2** and **3**).

CuTS is initially treated nonoperatively for about 3 to 6 months with active rest. A night splint in relative elbow extension, an elbow pad during the day, avoidance of aggravating activities (eg, triceps extension exercise, prolonged elbow flexion, and

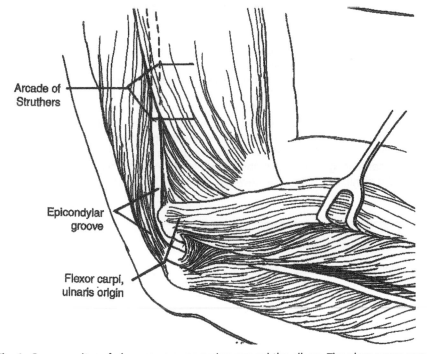

Arcade of Struthers

Epicondylar groove

Flexor carpi, ulnaris origin

Fig. 1. Common sites of ulnar nerve compression around the elbow. The ulnar nerve passes from the anterior to the posterior compartment through the arcade of Struthers (a fibrous sheath). It then passes between the medial epicondyle of the humerus and the olecranon in the epicondylar groove. It then passes between the 2 heads of the FCU and proceeds down the forearm under the deep surface of the FCU. (*From* Hentz VR, Chase RA. Hand surgery: a clinical atlas. Philadelphia: WB Saunders; 2001. Fig. 3-23, p. 263; with permission.)

Table 1	
Testing ulnar-innervated muscles distal to the cubital tunnel	
Muscle	**Test**
FDP to ulnar 2 digits	Resisted distal interphalangeal joint (DIP) flexion with proximal interphalangeal (PIP) joint extension
FCU	Resisted wrist flexion and ulnar deviation
Intrinsic first dorsal interossei strength	Resisted index finger abduction
Abductor digiti minimi (hypothenar muscles)	Resisted small finger abduction

repetitive elbow flexion and extension), and nonsteroidal antiinflammatory drugs (NSAIDs) can help decrease symptoms. A stretching routine is established for the elbow, forearm, and wrist. Athletes with symptoms primarily during throwing should cease throwing until they are asymptomatic. At about 6 weeks, progressive isometric strengthening exercises commence as tolerated. Throwing athletes should focus on strengthening the dynamic stabilizers of the elbow. There is then a gradual return to sport-specific functions, for example, starting first with interval throwing.[14,15] The mechanics of throwing should be scrutinized and modified as necessary. The longer the duration and severity of symptoms, the less likely conservative management will adequately relieve symptoms.[12] In particular, athletes with valgus instability of the elbow have a high symptomatic recurrence rate on resumption of throwing.[7]

For those patients with recalcitrant CuTS, operative management is discussed, namely nerve decompression at the elbow via release of the arcuate ligament. Those with more advanced symptoms, including motor weakness, may be considered for operative intervention earlier. After decompression, the nerve can be left in place or transposed anteriorly. The transposition can be subcutaneous held in place with a sling/pulley fashioned from the subcutaneous tissue and fascia over the flexor/ pronator muscles (**Fig. 4**),[16–19] submuscular (beneath a detached flexor pronator mass), or intramuscular (entailing less trauma to the flexor pronator mass compared with the submuscular transposition). A limited medial epicondylectomy with or without anterior transposition of the nerve may also be performed.[20–23]

Studies comparing the results of these techniques, including 2 meta-analyses, have not found a significant difference between the procedures in terms of postoperative

Table 2	
Provocative testing of the ulnar nerve	
Test Name	**Positive Sign**
Froment sign	Interphalangeal joint of thumb and DIP of index finger flex when trying to hold onto a piece of paper between the thumb and index finger to compensate for weak intrinsics
Elbow flexion test	Full elbow flexion, forearm supination, and wrist extension; elicits numbness, tingling, and/or pain in the ulnar nerve distribution. The earlier the test becomes positive, the more severely the cubital tunnel is involved. Analogous to the Phalen test for carpal tunnel syndrome
Tinel sign	Percussion of the ulnar nerve at the elbow (tapping) elicits numbness or tingling in the ulnar distribution or an electrical sensation travelling down the ulnar forearm and hand

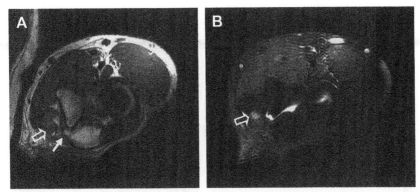

Fig. 2. (*A, B*) MRI of an elbow in a pitcher with valgus extension overload syndrome and ulnar neuritis. The axial T1-weighted (*A*) and T2-weighted (*B*) images show a swollen ulnar nerve (*open arrow*), with high T2 signal intensity. A posteromedial osteophyte is seen arising from the olecranon (*solid arrow*).

clinical outcomes or motor nerve conduction velocities.[24,25] All of these techniques have excellent results in the literature, and each have potential advantages and disadvantages (**Table 3**). In general, patients with symptoms lasting longer than 6 months have a worse prognosis.[26]

Regardless of the procedure, it is critical that the nerve be released adequately both proximally and distally. Furthermore, concomitant associated pathology (eg, valgus elbow instability and/or tearing or inflammation of the flexor pronator tendon origin) must be addressed to fully restore function and relieve pain. Simple decompression in situ and medial epicondylectomy are generally not preferred for throwers. The former may lead to nerve subluxation, and the latter jeopardizes the UCL and flexor origins.[7,27]

There are certain particularly noteworthy operative points that are highlighted here. After releasing the nerve, the elbow must be ranged intraoperatively to look for ulnar nerve subluxation or dislocation; if these occur, the nerve must be anteriorly transposed. The submuscular and intramuscular transpositions decrease the exposure of the nerve to direct pressure, which is particularly relevant in lean athletes or those subject to direct trauma (eg, wrestlers).[15] The most common cause of recurrence or persistence of CuTS after surgery is failure to release the nerve adequately at all potential sites of compression. The most common sites of persistent compression

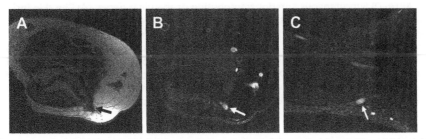

Fig. 3. (*A–C*) Axial T1-weighted (*A*), axial T2-weighted (*B*), and sagittal T2-weighted (*C*) images in a patient with ulnar neuritis showing focal swelling of the ulnar nerve (*arrow*), with high signal intensity on T2-weighted images.

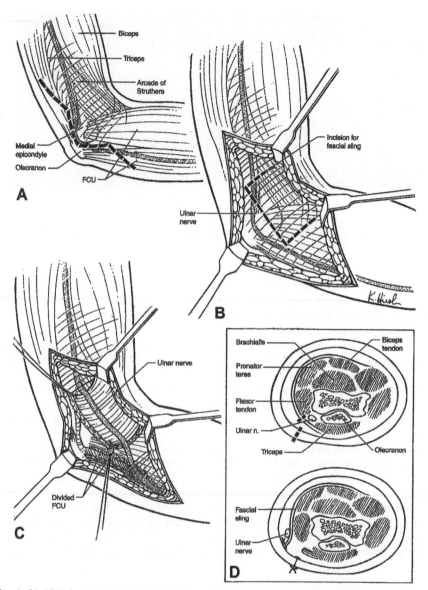

Fig. 4. (*A–D*) Subcutaneous anterior transposition of the ulnar nerve. (*A*) The skin incision can be either a curved line between the medial epicondyle and the olecranon or a lazy-M-shaped incision as pictured here. (*B*) After releasing the nerve at all possible sites of compression around the elbow, the nerve is transposed anteriorly and held there by a broad medial-based facial sling. (*C*) The ulnar nerve now lies on a broad fascial sheath, preventing it from displacing posteriorly. (*D*) The fascial shelf is anchored to the deep dermal layer once the optimal position of the nerve is determined. (*From* Hentz VR, Chase RA. Hand surgery: a clinical atlas. Philadelphia: WB Saunders; 2001. Fig. 3-26, p. 269; with permission.)

are the medial intermuscular septum, the arcade of Struthers, fibrous bands at the entrance or exit of the cubital tunnel, persistence or kinking at the Osborne arcuate ligament, fascial slings, and incomplete anterior transposition.[28] In a study of 100 patients who had a revision surgery for CuTS, the most common indications were

Table 3
Potential advantages and disadvantages of cubital tunnel decompression techniques

Technique	Advantages	Disadvantages: All Have Potential for Surgical Site Tenderness
Simple decompression	Preserves the flexor/pronator musculature Preserves the ulnar nerve blood supply	Nerve subluxation/dislocation Does not eliminate the tensile forces generated during elbow flexion 7% have persistent symptoms postoperatively (can be treated successfully with anterior submuscular transposition)
Subcutaneous transposition	Preserves the flexor/pronator musculature	Requires postoperative immobilization Nerve position superficial
Submuscular transposition	Nerve protected by muscle	Requires postoperative immobilization Disrupts flexor/pronator musculature
Medial epicondylectomy	Preserves the ulnar nerve blood supply	Local tenderness Nerve subluxation over the remaining epicondyle Flexor pronator weakness Flexion contracture Valgus instability caused by damage to the medial collateral ligament Subluxation of the ulnar nerve These risks are reduced with a partial medial epicondylectomy

Data from Brauer CA, Graham B. The surgical treatment of cubital tunnel syndrome: a decision analysis. J Hand Surg Eur Vol 2007;32(6):654–62.

increased ulnar nerve symptoms (55 patients) and pain in the medial antebrachial cutaneous nerve (MABCN) distribution (55 patients). The most common operative findings during the revision were MABCN neuroma (73 patients) and a distal kink of the ulnar nerve (57 patients).[29]

During the subcutaneous transposition, care must be taken when creating the sling tethering the nerve anteriorly as the sling itself can cause severe ulnar neuropathy. Release of a compressive sling often results in pain relief but incomplete sensory and motor recovery. Recurrent cubital tunnel syndrome is most often addressed by submuscular anterior transposition of the nerve.[17,29,30] If a patient with CuTS has an anconeus epitrochlearis muscle and no other identifiable causes of the neuropathy, simple excision of the muscle and release of any other tissue constraining the cubital tunnel relieve symptoms even without anterior transposition of the nerve.[5,31]

After the procedure, the elbow is immobilized in a position that minimizes tension on the nerve; usually a posterior splint in 60° of flexion with the forearm in neutral. In a study of subcutaneous transposition, the group immobilized in a long arm cast for 2 to 3 weeks postoperatively returned to work at an average of 30 days postoperatively, whereas those who had a soft dressing and were allowed immediate active range of motion (ROM) returned to work at an average of 9.6 days ($P = .002$).[18] Therapy is begun 1 week postoperatively, beginning with ROM, then isometric strengthening. The most difficult challenge is often achieving full elbow extension with forearm supination. Resistive training begins at 6 weeks postoperatively. Guided throwing programs begin at 8 weeks postoperatively. At 12 weeks postoperatively, restrictions are usually lifted.[15]

There are a few reports focusing on athletes with CuTS. In a retrospective study of 20 athletes (21 elbows) treated with subcutaneous transposition of the ulnar nerve, athletes returned to full activity at an average of 12.6 months (range 6–43 months). One patient required a second operation: neurolysis of the MABCN.[19] In a study of 15 throwing athletes treated with partial epicondylectomy and anterior subcutaneous transposition of the nerve, all had full strength and would have the surgery again. Fourteen were very satisfied, and 14 returned to throwing at an average of 7.4 months after surgery at their preinjury level or higher.[12]

We prefer a subcutaneous anterior transposition for throwers, even if they are lean, because of concern about detaching the flexor pronator origin and its effects on rehabilitation in these athletes. The flexor pronator mass is particularly important for throwers because it protects their UCL. We reserve submuscular anterior transposition for revision cases.

RADIAL NERVE ENTRAPMENT

The radial nerve (comprised of C5–T1 nerve roots from the posterior cord of the brachial plexus) travels through the radial tunnel at the lateral elbow. The radial tunnel is a 5-cm stretch over the anterior aspect of the proximal radius, starting just proximal to the capitellum and extending to the proximal edge of the supinator. Proximal to the supinator arch, the radial nerve divides into the sensory superficial branch of the radial nerve (SBRN) and the deep motor posterior interosseous nerve (PIN). The PIN then passes deep to the superficial portion of the supinator.

Although there are 5 classic sites of radial nerve compression in the radial tunnel, a variety of entities can compress the radial nerve at or near the elbow, causing 2 distinct entities: radial tunnel syndrome (RTS) or posterior interosseous nerve syndrome (PINS) (**Boxes 2** and **3**). RTS is purely a pain syndrome; there are no definitive objective clinical signs, NCSs are normal, and only 8% of patients have

Box 2
Classic sites of radial nerve compression in the radial tunnel (pneumonic: FREAS)
1. *F*ibrous bands of the radiocapitellar joint
2. *R*adial recurrent leash of blood vessels overlying the nerve (leash of Henry)
3. *E*xtensor carpi radialis brevis (ECRB)
4. *A*rcade of Frohse (most common site of entrapment)
5. *S*upinator proximal fascia and/or distal border

abnormalities of the PIN on EMG.[32] Any motor weakness is believed to be caused by pain rather than issues with muscle innervation. Patients often have nocturnal pain, awakening them from sleep. RTS may be caused by intermittent or dynamic compression of the PIN in the proximal forearm caused by repeated stressful pronation and supination. Athletes at particular risk for RTS are swimmers, tennis players, Frisbee players, and powerlifters.[33] An injection of a corticosteroid adjacent to the PIN at the level of the proximal radius may be helpful in establishing the diagnosis. The addition of a short-acting local anesthetic to the injection confirms accurate injection placement when there is a resulting PIN palsy.[34,35]

Chronic lateral elbow pain without motor weakness may be RTS or lateral epicondylitis (LE). There are several features that help distinguish the 2 entities, but the differences are often subtle (**Table 4**).[36,37] There is significant overlap between the 2 entities in terms of response to provocative maneuvers. Some argue that recalcitrant LE is actually RTS, whereas others argue that the 2 conditions may actually be an integrated pathology because the supinator and extensor carpi radialis brevis (ECRB) both produce tensile forces on the common extensor origins and put pressure onto the radial tunnel.[38]

PINS presents with distinct motor weakness, including finger extensor weakness (finger drop) and, to a lesser degree, wrist extensor weakness. PINS patients do not typically complain of pain, and, when pain is present, it is not their chief complaint.

Box 3
Other causes of radial nerve compression at or near the elbow
Rheumatoid synovitis/synovial cysts
Ganglion cysts
Periosteal lipoma of the proximal radius
Myxoma
Intracapsular chondroma
Synovial chondromatosis
Pseudogout
Brachiocephalic arteriovenous fistula
Synovial hemangioma
Tuberculous arthritis
Data from Mileti J, Largacha M, O'Driscoll SW. Radial tunnel syndrome caused by ganglion cyst: treatment by arthroscopic cyst decompression. Arthroscopy 2004;20(5):e39–44.

Table 4
Characteristics of RTS and LE

Characteristic	RTS	LE
Frequency	Rare (2% of all peripheral nerve compressions of the upper limb)	Common cause of lateral elbow pain
Cause	Compression of the radial nerve	Caused by overuse of the extensor and supinator muscles
Characteristic patient	Anybody with repetitive, stressful pronation and supination, eg, tennis players, Frisbee players, swimmers, powerlifters	Tennis players
Pain location	Pain over the neck of the radius and lateral aspect of the proximal forearm over the extensor muscles themselves (distal to where the pain is located in LE)	Pain and tenderness over the lateral epicondyle and immediately distal to it (at the origin of the extensor muscles)
Pain radiation	Pain can radiate proximally and (more commonly) distally	Usually localized without radiation
Provocative tests (much overlap between the 2 entities)	Pain with resisted extension of the middle finger with the forearm pronated and the elbow extended. Pain with resisted forearm supination with the elbow fully extended	Pain with resisted wrist extension or elbow supination with the elbow extended. Pain with forceful wrist flexion or forearm pronation

PINS is caused by continuous or intermittent compression of the PIN in the radial tunnel.[36,39]

Both RTS and PINS are most often initially treated nonoperatively with rest, NSAIDs, immobilization, and forearm splinting or bracing. However, patients with an identifiable source of compression (eg, a ganglion or lipoma within the radial tunnel) may be candidates for early surgical excision of the mass.[40] If PIN palsy persists, surgical release is an option (**Fig. 5**). In 1996, a decompression study reported motor recovery in 24 of 25 (96%) patients with PINS at minimum 2-month follow-up.[41] When there are motor deficits present, timing of surgery may affect outcomes (ie, earlier decompression is advantageous), and a delay in decompression of more than 18 months from onset of weakness may result in fibrosis of PIN-innervated muscles, making tendon transfers the only viable option.[34]

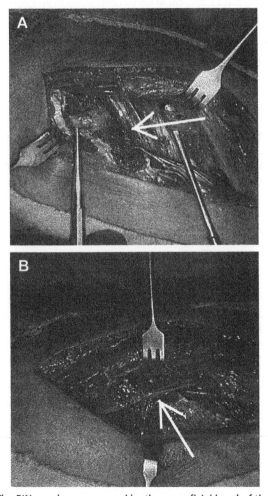

Fig. 5. (*A, B*) (*A*) The PIN may be compressed by the superficial head of the supinator, particularly at its proximal edge (the arcade of Frohse as indicated by the arrow). (*B*) Release of the superficial head of the supinator may decompress the PIN (*arrow*). (*From* Hentz VR, Chase RA. Hand surgery: a clinical atlas. Philadelphia: WB Saunders; 2001. Fig. 3-31, p. 280; with permission.)

Patients with RTS should avoid elbow extension, forearm pronation, and wrist flexion. If symptoms persist despite activity modification, an injection of lidocaine and triamcinolone has been shown to resolve RTS pain in 16 of 25 (64%) patients at minimum 6-month follow-up.[42] Recalcitrant cases are treated by open decompression at all possible sites of compression, but the outcome of neurolysis is unpredictable.[32,43] In 2008, a systematic review of observational studies (there are no randomized control trials) of radial tunnel release for RTS found effectiveness rates of 67% to 92% and patient satisfaction rates of 40% to 83%.[39] In 2009, a study of patients with RTS reported that the success rate of PIN decompression alone (most common technique) varies from 10% to 95%; success of decompressing both the PIN and the SBRN ranges from 67% to 92% (3 studies), and decompression of just the SBRN resulted in patient satisfaction in 11 of 12 patients (92%).[44] Risks of PIN decompression include damage to the PIN and iatrogenic extensor weakness from ECRB release. Coexisting LE and other nerve compression syndromes are associated with lower success rates.[45]

The focus of the first 3 weeks postoperatively is regaining full elbow ROM. Massage is used to desensitize the site, and the therapist supervises nerve-gliding exercises. At 3 weeks postoperatively, gentle resistive exercises are initiated. There is also a focus on stretching the ECRB and extensor digitorum communis (EDC) muscles (ie, elbow extended, forearm pronated, and wrist flexed). At 6 weeks postoperatively, strengthening of the wrist, elbow, and forearm starts progressing from isometrics, to concentrics, and then to eccentrics. Plyometric activities (eg, ball tossing) are used to incorporate the entire upper extremity. Return to sporting activity is begun only after ROM and strength have been fully restored.[15,38]

We have had good success with decompression of the PIN, particularly when an anatomic site of compression or mass effect (eg, a ganglion) is detected. We rarely operate on RTS in athletes because of the unpredictable results of this procedure.

PRONATOR SYNDROME

Pronator syndrome (also called high median nerve compression) involves compression of the median nerve (comprised of nerve roots C5–T1, formed by the blending of the lateral and medial cords of the brachial plexus). The nerve crosses anterior to the elbow, beneath the bicipital aponeurosis and superficial to the brachialis muscle. It runs medial and parallel to the brachial artery. It passes between the humeral (superficial) and ulnar (deep) heads of the pronator teres muscle and then under the fibrous aponeurotic arch of the flexor digitorum superficialis (FDS) (**Fig. 6**). The median nerve innervates the pronator teres, flexor carpi radialis (FCR), palmaris longus (PL), and FDS.

The median nerve is most commonly entrapped at 4 sites: the ligament of Struthers (originates at the supracondylar process and inserts on the medial epicondyle), the lacertus fibrosis (bicipital aponeurosis), the pronator teres muscle, and the proximal arch of the FDS. The most frequent cause of pronator syndrome is dynamic compression of the nerve between the 2 heads of the pronator teres muscle, exacerbated by forearm pronation and elbow extension. Sports that entail repetitive forceful pronation and supination (eg, pitching, rowing, weight training, and racquet sports) can cause pronator syndrome. The FDS may compress the median nerve in sports that entail gripping (eg, archery).[46]

Other causes of compression include extreme proximal forearm musculature hypertrophy in athletes, elbow fractures and dislocations, an accessory head of the flexor pollicis longus (FPL) (Gantzer muscle), a crossing radial artery and/or vein, and

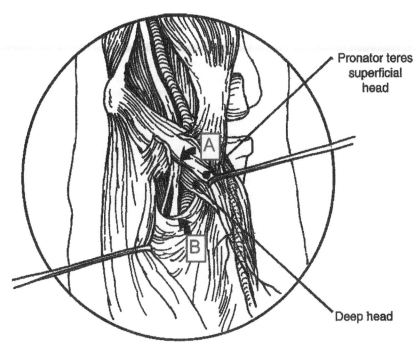

Pronator teres
superficial
head

Deep head

Fig. 6. The median nerve passes between the 2 heads of the pronator teres (*arrow A*). The anterior interosseous branch of the median nerve then passes deep to the FDS (*arrow B*). Both the pronator teres and the leading edge of the FDS are potential sites of median nerve compression. (*From* Hentz VR, Chase RA. Hand surgery: a clinical atlas. Philadelphia: WB Saunders; 2001. Figure 3-43, p. 306; with permission.)

space-occupying lesions (eg, nerve sheath tumors, ganglions, bursae). The median nerve can also be directly compressed in sports (eg, gymnastics) that entail maneuvers or equipment that places significant tension on the forearm musculature. Motorcycle distance racers may develop pronator syndrome as a result of the repetitive flexor contraction needed to control the brake lever.[47]

Pronator syndrome is a challenging diagnosis because many of the symptoms are activity-related and electrodiagnostic testing is often negative. The history and physical examination are therefore critical for an accurate diagnosis. Patients may complain of vague aching pain in the volar aspect of their elbow and forearm, exacerbated by activities requiring repetitive grasping and/or pronation. The most common physical examination finding is tenderness over the pronator muscle mass. One should look for fullness or a mass in anterior elbow. There may be tenderness to palpation along the median nerve in the forearm. Patients rarely have weakness, but it is subtle when present. Patients may have paresthesias of the palmar side of their radial digits with repetitive forearm pronation/supination, but not with elbow flexion and extension. Resistance to forearm pronation or flexion of just the middle and ring finger PIP joints elicits pain.[48]

Provocative tests may help localize the site of compression: active supination against resistance with the elbow hyperflexed (compression at the lacertus fibrosis), resisted forearm pronation followed by elbow extension (compression at the pronator teres), and resisted flexion of the long finger with the other fingers held in hyperextension (compression by the FDS).[46] An MRI from the distal one-third of the arm down to the proximal two-thirds of the forearm may be performed to look for causes of compression.

It is important to rule out carpal tunnel syndrome (CTS, entrapment of the median nerve at the wrist). Pronator syndrome is sometimes diagnosed after a carpal tunnel release has failed to relieve the symptoms. CTS is much more common than pronator syndrome, does not present with pain in the forearm, and often presents with nocturnal symptoms (which is rarely present in pronator syndrome). Patients with pronator syndrome may have numbness in the thenar eminence (palmar cutaneous branch of the median nerve) that is not seen in CTS patients because this branch does not pass through the carpal tunnel. Thenar atrophy indicates CTS but is rare in pronator syndrome. A positive Tinel sign at the wrist and a positive Phalen test support the diagnosis of CTS. Ultimately, cortisone injections at the carpal tunnel and the pronator at different times helps confirm the correct diagnosis.[46]

Pronator syndrome must also be differentiated from anterior interosseous nerve (AIN) syndrome (AINS). About 2 to 5 cm distal to the medial epicondyle, the median nerve gives off the AIN, which then travels down the forearm along the interosseous membrane, supplying the radial half of the FDP, the FPL, and the pronator quadratus (PQ). AINS patients do not have sensory symptoms but may have gross weakness that does not occur with pronator syndrome. Though NCSs and EMGs are not usually helpful in confirming pronator syndrome, these studies can exclude impaired nerve conduction at the wrist level (CTS) and denervation of muscles innervated by the AIN (AINS).[49] An MRI scan is not usually ordered, but may show increased fluid signal within and around the nerve (**Fig. 7**).

Conservative management of pronator syndrome entails rest from repetitive gripping and pronation activities. Equipment, athletic positions, and upper body mechanics should be analyzed and modified as necessary. NSAIDs, oral steroids, and/or local steroid injections may also help. The elbow can be splinted in 90° of flexion, the forearm in neutral to slight pronation, and the wrist in neutral to slight volar flexion.

The key to operative treatment is release of all 4 possible sites of median nerve entrapment. After the procedure, the elbow is placed in a posterior split at 60° to 70° of elbow flexion and 30° to 40° of pronation. Almost immediately, the therapist begins gentle active ROM of the elbow, then light resistive exercises at 3 to 4 weeks (isometrics and proximal/distal muscle strengthening) with an emphasis on

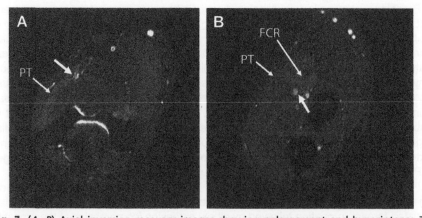

Fig. 7. (*A, B*) Axial inversion recovery images showing enlargement and hyperintense T2 signal within the median nerve (*arrow*) at the level of the medial epicondyle (*A*), and in the midforearm (*B*). PT, pronator teres; FCR, flexor carpi radialis.

strengthening forearm flexor muscles. At 6 to 8 weeks postoperatively, sports-specific exercises are introduced and advanced as tolerated.[15]

Medial Antebrachial Cutaneous Neuropathy

The MABCN (comprised of T1 and T2 nerve roots from the medial cord or the lower trunk of the brachial plexus) is a purely sensory nerve, innervating the medial aspect of the elbow and forearm. It divides into an anterior and posterior branch about 14.5 cm proximal to the medial humeral epicondyle. It may then again subdivide, and there are often between 1 and 3 anterior branches that cross the elbow.[50] MABCN neuropathy may be caused by steroid injection for medial epicondylitis, venipuncture, cubital tunnel release, UCL reconstruction, elbow arthroscopy, fracture fixation, tumor excision, arthrolysis, removal or insertion of implantable hormonal contraceptives, a lipoma, or repeated minor trauma (eg, tennis). Patients present with pain, numbness, and/or dysesthesia in the anteromedial elbow and the medial forearm.[51] In nontraumatic cases, a local corticosteroid injection may result in rapid lasting relief.[52] If the nerve has been cut, a microsurgical epineural nerve coaptation with 10-0 Ethilon may be attempted. Otherwise, the proximal end of the cut nerve should be cauterized, transposed proximally, and buried into muscle. If a persistent painful neuroma forms, it should be resected and the proximal stump should be buried into muscle.[50,53,54]

Lateral Antebrachial Cutaneous Neuropathy

The lateral antebrachial cutaneous nerve (LABCN) is the terminal sensory branch of the musculocutaneous nerve (comprised of C5 and C6 nerve roots from the lateral cord of the brachial plexus). It emerges from the lateral margin of the biceps (where it can be entrapped) about 2 to 5 cm proximal to the elbow flexion crease, then pierces the brachial fascia (another potential point of entrapment), and becomes subcutaneous. Entrapment neuropathy of the LABCN is an uncommon cause of anterolateral elbow pain.[55,56] LABCN entrapment at the lateral biceps edge has been described in throwing athletes and is sometimes termed the Bassett lesion.[57,58] Neuropraxia of the LABCN is not uncommon after retraction in single-incision distal biceps repair; the surgeon must be cognizant of its path to avoid more serious injury.

Patients present with paresthesias or burning dysesthesia along the volar lateral forearm. On physical examination, symptoms are induced by forced pronation and extension (mimicking ball release during a throw) of the elbow. There may be a positive Tinel sign just lateral to the biceps tendon. LABCN entrapment can be differentiated from LE and RTS by injecting the lateral margin of the biceps about 2 to 4 cm proximal to the elbow flexion crease with a local anesthetic.

Few patients respond to nonoperative management (eg, rest, NSAIDs, activity modification, a splint blocking full elbow extension). Surgical treatment yields excellent results and entails releasing the nerve completely proximally (at the lateral margin of the biceps) and distally (at the bicipital aponeurosis). The nerve is found by extension and pronation of the elbow. A triangular wedge of biceps aponeurosis may also be removed along the lateral edge of the biceps. Postoperative management includes splinting in 90° of flexion for 5 to 7 days with a return to full activities in 2 to 3 weeks.[59–62]

SUMMARY

The ulnar, radial, median, medial antebrachial cutaneous, and LABCNs all cross the elbow joint and are subject to compression or traction in that region. CuTS (ulnar nerve) is by far the most common neuropathy about the elbow. Athletes in particular may place high stresses on their elbow, leading to sources of traction (eg, UCL laxity) and compression (eg, hypertrophic muscles). Each neuropathy causes a distinct syndrome based on the anatomy and innervation of that particular nerve. The motor sequelae of these conditions may be debilitating for an athlete dependent on fine motor control and explosive strength; pain may also severely limit athletic function. Electrodiagnostic studies are often unreliable, and so the history and physical examination are of paramount importance in the work-up. Nonoperative and operative treatments for athletes must take into account the specific demands of their sports.

ACKNOWLEDGMENTS

The authors thank Kathryn J. Stevens, MD (Department of Radiology, Stanford University Medical Center) for providing and annotating the MRI images included in this article.

REFERENCES

1. O'Driscoll SW, Horii E, Carmichael SW, et al. The cubital tunnel and ulnar neuropathy. J Bone Joint Surg Br 1991;73(4):613–7.
2. Norkus SA, Meyers MC. Ulnar neuropathy of the elbow. Sports Med 1994;17(3): 189–99.
3. Patel VV, Heidenreich FP Jr, Bindra RR, et al. Morphologic changes in the ulnar nerve at the elbow with flexion and extension: a magnetic resonance imaging study with 3-dimensional reconstruction. J Shoulder Elbow Surg 1998;7(4):368–74.
4. Matsuura S, Kojima T, Kinoshita Y. Cubital tunnel syndrome caused by abnormal insertion of triceps brachii muscle. J Hand Surg Br 1994;19(1):38–9.
5. Boero S, Senes FM, Catena N. Pediatric cubital tunnel syndrome by anconeus epitrochlearis: a case report. J Shoulder Elbow Surg 2009;18(2):e21–3.
6. Dahners LE, Wood FM. Anconeus epitrochlearis, a rare cause of cubital tunnel syndrome: a case report. J Hand Surg Am 1984;9(4):579–80.
7. Cummins CA, Schneider DS. Peripheral nerve injuries in baseball players. Phys Med Rehabil Clin N Am 2009;20(1):175–93, x.
8. Ozbek A, Bamac B, Budak F, et al. Nerve conduction study of ulnar nerve in volleyball players. Scand J Med Sci Sports 2006;16(3):197–200.
9. Treihaft MM. Neurologic injuries in baseball players. Semin Neurol 2000;20(2):187–93.
10. McGowan AJ. The results of transposition of the ulnar nerve for traumatic ulnar neuritis. J Bone Joint Surg Br 1950;32(3):293–301.
11. Buchthal F, Rosenfalck A, Trojaborg W. Electrophysiological findings in entrapment of the median nerve at wrist and elbow. J Neurol Neurosurg Psychiatry 1974;37(3):340–60.
12. Grana W. Medial epicondylitis and cubital tunnel syndrome in the throwing athlete. Clin Sports Med 2001;20(3):541–8.
13. Okamoto M, Abe M, Shirai H, et al. Diagnostic ultrasonography of the ulnar nerve in cubital tunnel syndrome. J Hand Surg Br 2000;25(5):499–502.
14. Cain EL Jr, Dugas JR, Wolf RS, et al. Elbow injuries in throwing athletes: a current concepts review. Am J Sports Med 2003;31(4):621–35.
15. Badia A, Stennett C. Sports-related injuries of the elbow. J Hand Ther 2006;19(2): 206–26.
16. Hashiguchi H, Ito H, Sawaizumi T. Stabilized subcutaneous transposition of the ulnar nerve. Int Orthop 2003;27(4):232–4.

17. Caputo AE, Watson HK. Subcutaneous anterior transposition of the ulnar nerve for failed decompression of cubital tunnel syndrome. J Hand Surg Am 2000; 25(3):544–51.

18. Black BT, Barron OA, Townsend PF, et al. Stabilized subcutaneous ulnar nerve transposition with immediate range of motion. Long-term follow-up. J Bone Joint Surg Am 2000;82(11):1544–51.

19. Rettig AC, Ebben JR. Anterior subcutaneous transfer of the ulnar nerve in the athlete. Am J Sports Med 1993;21(6):836–9 [discussion: 839–40].

20. Muermans S, De Smet L. Partial medial epicondylectomy for cubital tunnel syndrome: outcome and complications. J Shoulder Elbow Surg 2002;11(3):248–52.

21. Popa M, Dubert T. Treatment of cubital tunnel syndrome by frontal partial medial epicondylectomy. A retrospective series of 55 cases. J Hand Surg Br 2004;29(6): 563–7.

22. Gobel F, Musgrave DS, Vardakas DG, et al. Minimal medial epicondylectomy and decompression for cubital tunnel syndrome. Clin Orthop Relat Res 2001;393: 228–36.

23. Efstathopoulos DG, Themistocleous GS, Papagelopoulos PJ, et al. Outcome of partial medial epicondylectomy for cubital tunnel syndrome. Clin Orthop Relat Res 2006;444:134–9.

24. Zlowodzki M, Chan S, Bhandari M, et al. Anterior transposition compared with simple decompression for treatment of cubital tunnel syndrome. A meta-analysis of randomized, controlled trials. J Bone Joint Surg Am 2007; 89(12):2591 8.

25. Macadam SA, Gandhi R, Bezuhly M, et al. Simple decompression versus anterior subcutaneous and submuscular transposition of the ulnar nerve for cubital tunnel syndrome: a meta-analysis. J Hand Surg Am 2008;33(8):1314.e1–12.

26. Charles YP, Coulet B, Rouzaud JC, et al. Comparative clinical outcomes of submuscular and subcutaneous transposition of the ulnar nerve for cubital tunnel syndrome. J Hand Surg Am 2009;34(5):866–74.

27. Aldridge JW, Bruno RJ, Strauch RJ, et al. Nerve entrapment in athletes. Clin Sports Med 2001;20(1):95–122.

28. Kleinman WB. Revision ulnar neuroplasty. Hand Clin 1994;10(3):461–77.

29. Mackinnon SE, Novak CB. Operative findings in reoperation of patients with cubital tunnel syndrome. Hand (N Y) 2007;2(3):137–43.

30. Polatsch DB, Bong MR, Rokito AS. Severe ulnar neuropathy after subcutaneous transposition in a collegiate tennis player. Am J Orthop 2002;31(11):643–6.

31. Masear VR, Hill JJ Jr, Cohen SM. Ulnar compression neuropathy secondary to the anconeus epitrochlearis muscle. J Hand Surg Am 1988;13(5):720–4.

32. Jebson PJ, Engber WD. Radial tunnel syndrome: long-term results of surgical decompression. J Hand Surg Am 1997;22(5):889–96.

33. Dickerman RD, Stevens QE, Cohen AJ, et al. Radial tunnel syndrome in an elite power athlete: a case of direct compressive neuropathy. J Peripher Nerv Syst 2002;7(4):229–32.

34. Dang AC, Rodner CM. Unusual compression neuropathies of the forearm, part I: radial nerve. J Hand Surg Am 2009;34(10):1906–14.

35. Ritts GD, Wood MB, Linscheid RL. Radial tunnel syndrome. A ten-year surgical experience. Clin Orthop Relat Res 1987;219:201–5.

36. Campbell WW, Landau ME. Controversial entrapment neuropathies. Neurosurg Clin N Am 2008;19(4):597–608, vi–vii.

37. Papanastasiou S, Ikram MS. A tried and tested surgical technique for recurrent radial tunnel syndrome. J Plast Reconstr Aesthet Surg 2009;62(5):e83–4.

38. Henry M, Stutz C. A unified approach to radial tunnel syndrome and lateral tendinosis. Tech Hand Up Extrem Surg 2006;10(4):200–5.
39. Huisstede B, Miedema HS, van Opstal T, et al. Interventions for treating the radial tunnel syndrome: a systematic review of observational studies. J Hand Surg Am 2008;33(1):72–8.
40. Mileti J, Largacha M, O'Driscoll SW. Radial tunnel syndrome caused by ganglion cyst: treatment by arthroscopic cyst decompression. Arthroscopy 2004;20(5): e39–44.
41. Hashizume H, Nishida K, Nanba Y, et al. Non-traumatic paralysis of the posterior interosseous nerve. J Bone Joint Surg Br 1996;78(5):771–6.
42. Sarhadi NS, Korday SN, Bainbridge LC. Radial tunnel syndrome: diagnosis and management. J Hand Surg Br 1998;23(5):617–9.
43. Sotereanos DG, Varitimidis SE, Giannakopoulos PN, et al. Results of surgical treatment for radial tunnel syndrome. J Hand Surg Am 1999;24(3):566–70.
44. Bolster MA, Bakker XR. Radial tunnel syndrome: emphasis on the superficial branch of the radial nerve. J Hand Surg Eur Vol 2009;34(3):343–7.
45. Lee JT, Azari K, Jones NF. Long term results of radial tunnel release–the effect of co-existing tennis elbow, multiple compression syndromes and workers' compensation. J Plast Reconstr Aesthet Surg 2008;61(9):1095–9.
46. Rehak DC. Pronator syndrome. Clin Sports Med 2001;20(3):531–40.
47. Goubier JN, Saillant G. Chronic compartment syndrome of the forearm in competitive motor cyclists: a report of two cases. Br J Sports Med 2003;37(5): 452–3 [discussion: 453–4].
48. Bencardino JT, Rosenberg ZS. Entrapment neuropathies of the shoulder and elbow in the athlete. Clin Sports Med 2006;25(3):465–87, vi–vii.
49. Werner CO, Rosen I, Thorngren KG. Clinical and neurophysiologic characteristics of the pronator syndrome. Clin Orthop Relat Res 1985;197:231–6.
50. Lowe JB 3rd, Maggi SP, Mackinnon SE. The position of crossing branches of the medial antebrachial cutaneous nerve during cubital tunnel surgery in humans. Plast Reconstr Surg 2004;114(3):692–6.
51. Yildiz N, Ardic F. A rare cause of forearm pain: anterior branch of the medial antebrachial cutaneous nerve injury: a case report. J Brachial Plex Peripher Nerve Inj 2008;3:10.
52. Seror P. Forearm pain secondary to compression of the medial antebrachial cutaneous nerve at the elbow. Arch Phys Med Rehabil 1993;74(5):540–2.
53. Wechselberger G, Wolfram D, Pulzl P, et al. Nerve injury caused by removal of an implantable hormonal contraceptive. Am J Obstet Gynecol 2006;195(1): 323–6.
54. Nash C, Staunton T. Focal brachial cutaneous neuropathy associated with Norplant use: suggests careful consideration of the recommended site for inserting contraceptive implants. J Fam Plann Reprod Health Care 2001;27(3): 155–6.
55. Narasanagi SS. Compression of lateral cutaneous nerve of forearm. Neurol India 1972;20(4):224–5.
56. Hale BR. Handbag paraesthesia. Lancet 1976;2(7983):470.
57. Davidson JJ, Bassett FH 3rd, Nunley JA 2nd. Musculocutaneous nerve entrapment revisited. J Shoulder Elbow Surg 1998;7(3):250–5.
58. Bassett FH 3rd, Nunley JA. Compression of the musculocutaneous nerve at the elbow. J Bone Joint Surg Am 1982;64(7):1050–2.
59. Gillingham BL, Mack GR. Compression of the lateral antebrachial cutaneous nerve by the biceps tendon. J Shoulder Elbow Surg 1996;5(4):330–2.

60. Naam NH, Massoud HA. Painful entrapment of the lateral antebrachial cutaneous nerve at the elbow. J Hand Surg Am 2004;29(6):1148–53.
61. Dailiana ZH, Roulot E, Le Viet D. Surgical treatment of compression of the lateral antebrachial cutaneous nerve. J Bone Joint Surg Br 2000;82(3):420–3.
62. Alberta FG, Elattrache NS. Diagnosis and treatment of distal biceps and anterior elbow pain in throwing athletes. Sports Med Arthrosc 2008;16(3):118–23.

Pediatric Sports Elbow Injuries

R. Michael Greiwe, MD, Comron Saifi, MS,
Christopher S. Ahmad, MD*

KEYWORDS

• Capitellar osteochondritis dissecans • Panner disease
• Medial epicondyle apophysitis • Persistent olecranon physis
• Medial collateral ligament

Our youth athletes are now exposed to exceptional performance demands, which has resulted in increased training at young ages. Approximately 35 million children and adolescents participate in sports annually in the United States and more than 2 million kids participate in Little League activities. Among children younger than 15 years, more than 3.5 million are treated for sports-related injuries. In particular, upper extremity and elbow injuries have increased with 20% to 40% of 9- to 12-year-old baseball players and 50% to 70% of adolescent players developing elbow pain annually.[1,2] Clearly, the elbow is vulnerable to injury in the youth athlete who participates in overhead or upper extremity weight-bearing sports such as gymnastics. Although fractures and dislocations commonly occur in collision sports, cartilage, subchondral bone, ligament, and apophyseal injuries occur from low-impact overuse sports. Specific injuries in the growing child are different compared with injuries in adults and this is even more pronounced in the skeletally immature elbow. Evaluation and management of elbow injuries in young athletes requires knowledge of the immature developing anatomy, injury pathophysiology, and established treatment algorithms for each diagnosis. Furthermore, risk factors contributing to elbow injuries must be recognized and prevention programs must be established.

ANATOMY

The elbow is a diarthrodial joint comprised of the distal humeral trochlea and capitellum, which articulate with the proximal ulna and radial head. Joint stability is produced by overall joint geometry, active muscle stabilizers, and passive ligamentous stabilizers. Congruent articular geometry imparts primary stability at elbow positions less than 20° and greater than 120° of flexion. Although articular geometry contributes to stability between 20 and 120°, the ulnar collateral ligament (UCL) complex is the

Columbia University Medical Center, Department of Orthopaedic Surgery, 622 West 168th Street, PH11-1130, New York, NY 10032, USA
* Corresponding author.
E-mail address: csa4@columbia.edu

Clin Sports Med 29 (2010) 677–703
doi:10.1016/j.csm.2010.06.010
0278-5919/10/$ – see front matter © 2010 Elsevier Inc. All rights reserved.

primary stabilizer to valgus force in this range. Valgus elbow stress is dynamically resisted by the flexor carpi ulnaris (FCU), flexor digitorum superficialis, and pronator teres.[3]

The UCL complex consists of an anterior bundle, posterior bundle, and transverse bundle.[4] The anterior bundle is the primary restraint to valgus stress and originates from the anteroinferior aspect of the medial epicondyle and inserts onto the sublime tubercle of the coronoid process. The anterior bundle is subdivided into anterior and posterior bands.[5] The UCL must withstand near-failure levels of tensile stress during the acceleration phase of the throwing motion.[4] Dynamic muscular stabilization prevents excessive valgus forces acting on the UCL. Electromyography studies indicate that pitchers with valgus instability have decreased flexor-pronator mass activity when pitching.[6] A cadaver study speculated that the FCU contributes to valgus elbow stability because of its anatomic position parallel to the UCL. Park and Ahmad[3] simulated muscle forces in cadavers and demonstrated that the flexor-pronator mass is an essential valgus stabilizer. That study determined the FCU as the primary stabilizer and the flexor digitorium superficialis as the secondary stabilizer.

The elbow joint is primarily cartilaginous in very young children with secondary ossification centers developing with further maturity. Growth at the elbow is primarily appositional through the apophyses, whereas 80% of longitudinal growth occurs at the proximal humerus. Knowledge of the age at which each ossification center appears helps differentiate normal anatomy from fractures and avulsions. The secondary ossification centers appear at the following ages: capitellum at 2 years old, radial head at 4 years old, medial (internal) epicondyle at 6 years old, trochlea at 7 years old, olecranon at 9 years old, and lateral (external) epicondyle at 10 years old.[7,8] The mnemonic CRITOE is popular to assist recall of the order of ossification. In girls the centers appear approximately 6 to 12 months before boys. By age 14 to 15 years in girls and 15 to 17 years in boys, all of the ossification centers fuse.

PITCHING BIOMECHANICS

Research is ongoing to better the understand the biomechanics of youth baseball pitching, which can also be extrapolated to other sports such as tennis, javelin, and volleyball, that produce a similar mechanism of valgus stress to the elbow. Overhead throwing can be broken down into 7 phases: windup, early cocking, late cocking, early acceleration, late acceleration, deceleration and follow-through (**Fig. 1**). During each phase, different stresses are produced on 3 major areas of the elbow. The valgus force at the elbow translates into tension on the medial aspect, compression on the lateral aspect, and shear in the posterior aspect (**Fig. 2**). The medial tensile forces are resisted by the UCL and flexor-pronator mass. The lateral compression forces are resisted by the radiocapitellar joint. The posterior shear force is resisted by the posteromedial tip of the olecranon, olecranon fossa, and trochlea.

Although the motion and kinematics of throwing have shown some similarities in children and adults, further research indicates marked differences.[9,10] Younger Little League players demonstrate slower hip rotation, slower trunk rotation, slower shoulder external rotation velocity, increased horizontal shoulder adduction during the cocking phase, less abduction in the acceleration phase, and overall less arm-body synchronization.[10] Increased joint forces and torques in a higher-level baseball pitcher are most likely to the result of increased muscle mass and strength.

Using video motion analysis, Limpisvasti[11] scrutinized 5 commonly taught pitching parameters: (1) leading with the pelvis in the windup phase; (2) hand on top of the ball

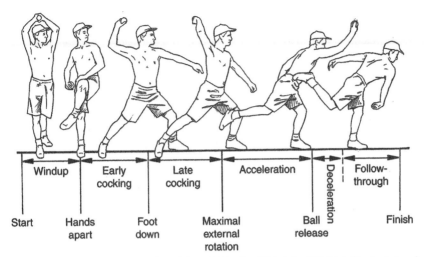

Fig. 1. Phases of pitching. (*Reproduced from* DiGiovine NM, Jobe FW, Pink M, et al. An electromyographic analysis of the upper extremity in pitching. J Shoulder Elbow Surg 1992;1:16; with permission.)

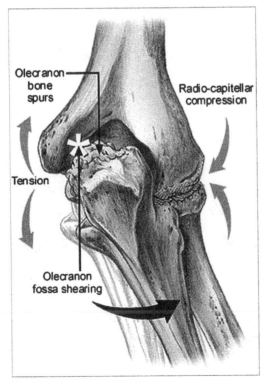

Fig. 2. Elbow biomechanics during the throwing motion. Valgus forces at the elbow result in tension in the medial structures, compression of lateral structures, and posteromedial shear. (*Reproduced from* Safran MR. Injury to the UCL: diagnosis and treatment. Sports Med Arthrosc Rev 2003;11:17; with permission.)

in early cocking (**Fig. 3**) and in late cocking; (3) shoulder closed (preventing opening up too soon) (**Fig. 4**); (4) the stride foot centered and pointing toward the home plate; and (5) elbow placed higher than hand. They found that adolescent pitchers (age 14–18 years) executed more parameters correctly than youth pitchers (age 9–13 years). Another study comparing Little League, adolescent, and college/professional pitchers, found that the younger Little League players generated slower trunk rotation, hip rotation, and shoulder external rotation velocity, had increased horizontal adduction in the cocking phase, less arm abduction during acceleration, and in general did not synchronize the arm motion with the body.[9] The valgus load and humeral internal rotation torque were significantly decreased when at least 3 parameters were performed correctly. This has even greater significance when one considers that joint forces and torque have been found to increase as pitchers mature, essentially doubling from the youth to the professional level.[9] Poor mechanics, with its concomitant unpredictable and pathologic stresses on the elbow, may culminate in injury as a youth pitcher grows and develops. Therefore, proper mechanics should be stressed as early in development as possible.

Biomechanical studies have estimated a maximum upper extremity acceleration of 500,000 degrees/s^2 and an angular velocity between 2300 and 5000 degrees/s during throwing in adults.[12–14] The anterior bundle of the UCL is primarily responsible for resisting the moments, estimated between 52 and 120 N m.[15,16] During pitching the UCL has been estimated to withstand 35 N m of torque[15] and 290 N of force.[16] A study by Ahmad and colleagues[17] determined the ultimate failure of the UCL to be 34 N m, approximately the demands of pitching. The adult thrower has dynamic stabilizing forces of the flexor digitorum superficialis (FDS) and FCU against valgus stress.[3] The adolescent thrower has a weak link of the medial epicondyle apophysis through which both the forces of the UCL and flexor-pronator mass act creating a risk of avulsion fractures.

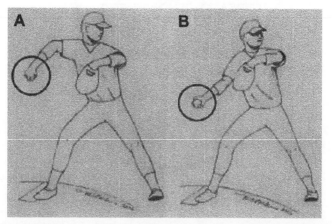

Fig. 3. The hand should stay above the elbow during throwing to decrease shoulder and elbow torques. (*A*) Proper hand position above the ball in late cocking. (*B*) Improper hand position below the ball before early acceleration. (*Reproduced from* Davis JT, Limpisvasti O, Fluhme D, et al. The effect of pitching biomechanics on the upper extremity in youth and adolescent baseball pitchers. Am J Sports Med 2009;37(8):1486; with permission.)

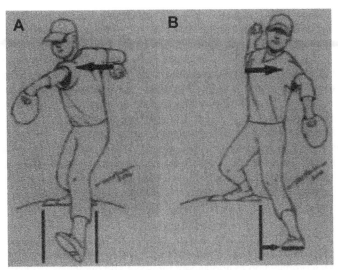

Fig. 4. The shoulder should stay closed to decrease elbow torque. (*A*) Shoulder stays closed in late cocking and early acceleration. (*B*) Shoulder open during late cocking and early acceleration. (*Reproduced from* Davis JT, Limpisvasti O, Fluhme D, et al. The effect of pitching biomechanics on the upper extremity in youth and adolescent baseball pitchers. Am J Sports Med 2009;37(8):1486; with permission.)

OVERUSE INJURIES

Overuse is becoming the most recognized factor influencing the alarming injury rates in young athletes. Most elbow injuries in youth athletes are related to repetitive overuse from overhead activities or elbow weight-bearing sports such as gymnastics. Depending on the nature of the patient's sport and their physiologic age, these injuries occur in predictable anatomic locations based on the biomechanics of throwing. Medial side injuries are related to chronic tension forces, the lateral side injuries are caused by repetitive compression forces, and posterior injuries are related to shear forces and repetitive abutment of the olecranon and the olecranon fossa. It is helpful to conceptually divide the elbow into 3 compartments based on the location of pain when constructing a differential diagnosis and treatment strategy.

LATERAL ELBOW INJURIES
Panner Disease

In 1927, Hans Panner described an osteochondrosis of the capitellum.[18] This osteo-chondrosis shares demographic, histologic, and radiographic features with Legg-Calvé-Perthes because the diseases affect boys less than 10 years of age, demonstrates abnormalities in endochondral ossification, and presents with evidence of fragmentation of an ossific nucleus.[19,20] Boys may be affected more than girls because of the delayed appearance and maturation of their secondary ossification centers and increased exposure to repetitive forces during childhood. However, this gender-specific feature may change as more young girls become involved in higher-risk athletic activities. Many theories exist to further explain the pathophysi-ology of Panner disease including disordered ossification from coagulation dyscrasias, endocrinopathies, and genetic factors. However, the current leading theory is that abnormal radiocapitellar compression during a vulnerable period of growth damages the posterior-based end-arterial supply to the capitellum compromising endochondral ossification.

Initial complaints are vague lateral elbow pain and stiffness. With prolonged symptoms, a 15 to 20° flexion contracture may develop. A slight effusion may be present and pain may be reproduced with extension and supination in combination with valgus load. Radiographs during the acute phase show fissuring and fragmentation of the capitellum. With time, radiographs return to normal corresponding to resolution of symptoms.

Panner disease has a natural history of symptom and pathology resolution. A period of immobilization is suggested for 1 to 3 weeks followed by mobilization and avoidance of repetitive elbow stress. When symptoms abate, a gradual return to repetitive stress may be instituted. If other joints are involved, a more comprehensive workup should be pursued including endocrine and genetic evaluations.

Osteochondritis Dissecans

Osteochondritis dissecans (OCD) is a noninflammatory degeneration of subchondral bone that has a predilection to adolescent throwers and gymnasts.[21] OCD commonly involves the capitellum and rarely involves the radial head as a primary location. Like Panner disease, the cause is not fully understood, and some investigators believe that OCD and Panner disease represent the same pathologic entity.[22,23] However, differences in age of onset and natural history fundamentally differentiate the lesions. In contrast to Panner disease, OCD develops in slightly older athletes aged 11 to 15 years, and the lesions can cause capitellar destruction.

The cause of OCD is theorized as a result of repetitive compressive forces generated when throwing, swinging a racquet, or performing activities of significant axial compression, such as gymnastics.[24,25] The theory is supported by evidence that overtraining in gymnastics and pitching results in a higher incidence of OCD.[25] In addition, poor blood supply may be a factor. The capitellum is supplied by 2 end-artery branches of the radial recurrent and interosseous recurrent arteries.[26] Local blood flow to the capitellum may be disrupted by both repetitive microtrauma or a single traumatic event leading to subchondral bone injury.[27,28]

Patients with OCD of the capitellum complain of activity-related pain and stiffness. Mechanical symptoms of locking or catching may indicate intraarticular loose bodies. Physical examination demonstrates tenderness over the radiocapitellar joint and commonly loss of 15 to 20° of extension. The active radiocapitellar compression test is positive for OCD lesions and elicits pain in the lateral compartment of the elbow when the patient pronates and supinates the forearm with the elbow in extension.

Anterioposterior radiographs in full extension and 45° of flexion, and lateral radiographs should be obtained when there is any suspicion for OCD. Radiographs may not demonstrate abnormality early in the disease process, but as the disease progresses, a focal anterolateral subchondral lucency is observed with surrounding sclerosis, named the crescent sign (**Fig. 5**).[29] Radiographic changes can persist for years.[30] Magnetic resonance imaging (MRI) is the best imaging tool, especially early in the disease process and should always be obtained. T1-weighted sequences demonstrate the early OCD lesion better than the T2 sequence, but T2 sequences establish fragment or perifragment enhancement with improved accuracy.[30] Unstable lesions are best demonstrated by MR arthrography. A pseudodefect is a sharp transition between the smooth articular surface of the posterior-inferior aspect of the capitellum and the rough nonarticular surface of the adjacent lateral epicondyle, and should not be confused with an OCD lesion.[31]

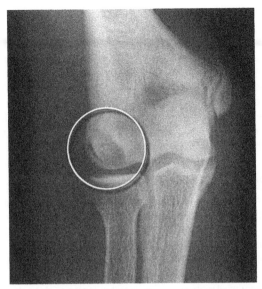

Fig. 5. Anterioposterior radiograph demonstrating an OCD lesion with surrounding sclerosis. (*Courtesy of* Center for Shoulder, Elbow and Sports Medicine at Columbia University.)

Classification and management of OCD lesions depend on 3 factors: the status of the capitellar growth plate, size and location of the lesion, and the nature and stability of the fragment. Arthroscopic and MRI grading systems correlate with each other, and can identify the stage of the lesion and guide treatment.[32] Several classifications systems have been described and some are cumbersome to use and guide treatment. We there therefore prefer to use a simple classification that is outlined in **Table 1**.

Type I: Stable Lesions

Type IA lesions are visualized only on the T1 MRI sequences. Arthroscopic evaluation demonstrates a normal cartilage surface. Patients are treated nonoperatively with cessation of activities that load the capitellum such as throwing, gymnastics, push-ups and weight lifting. The arm may be protected for 1 to 3 weeks in an elbow brace with intermittent range-of-motion exercises to prevent stiffness. Formal physical therapy following immobilization further prevents stiffness and when symptoms resolve, strengthening is initiated. Type IA lesions have an excellent prognosis with return to athletics expected by 4 to 6 months.

Table 1			
Classification of capitellar osteochondritis dissecans			
Type	**XR Findings**	**MRI Findings**	**Arthroscopic Findings**
IA	Normal	T1 signal	Normal
IB	Normal	T1 and T2 signal	Cartilage stable, soft
II	Radiolucent lesion	Rim-enhancing lesion	Loose flap
III	Crescent sign, radiolucent lesion with sclerotic rim	Osteochondral defect, loose bodies	Exposed bone, loose bodies

In type IB lesions, both MRI sequences are abnormal. Initially, patients should be treated similar to type IA lesions. Return to sport usually can be expected at 3 to 6 months. Follow-up radiographs and MRI scans should be obtained at 2- to 3-month intervals to track progress. If symptoms return, additional rest is mandated. With persistent refractory symptoms, pitchers may have to change positions and gymnasts may have to choose another sport. If after 3 to 6 months there is no improvement, surgery is indicated. During arthroscopy, the cartilage is intact, but soft because the subchondral bone is weakened. For lesions with a stable cartilage cap or only softening of the cartilage, retrograde or transarticular drilling with a 1.14-mm (0.045-in) smooth Kirschner wire is performed to stimulate healing.

Type II: Unstable or Partially Unstable Fragments

Type II lesions are unstable or partially unstable and show an enhancing rim surrounding the subchondral bone on MRI (**Fig. 6**). During an arthroscopic examination, the cartilage is fractured and the subchondral bone is unstable. The natural history of an unstable OCD is poor, especially if the lateral column is involved.[33] For completely unstable lesions greater than 5 mm, treatment options include debridement, debridement and drilling, osteochondral grafting, or fragment fixation. Lesion size and location govern treatment. For smaller lesions, debridement is preferred. Patients typically find immediate relief, but the development of early arthritis is common. Fragment fixation has been reported, but the healing potential of diseased subchondral bone and cartilage are unpredictable.[34–37] For large, radial head-engaging defects involving the lateral buttress of the capitellum, osteochondral grafting is considered. In the authors' opinion, if the decision must be made between osteochondral graft and fragment fixation, osteochondral graft provides more predictable results.

ElAttrache[38] and Ruch and colleagues[33] describe lateral extension of the lesion as a poor prognostic indicator. The lateral column of the capitellum supports large compressive forces, and lesions that do not involve a significant portion of the lateral

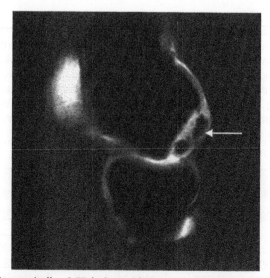

Fig. 6. MRI showing capitellar OCD lesion with associated loose body. (*Courtesy of* Center for Shoulder, Elbow and Sports Medicine at Columbia University.)

buttress of the capitellum and do not engage the radial head during arthroscopic examination (pronation and supination with the elbow in extension) are relatively protected and can be successfully treated with microfracture or drilling. However, if more than 6 to 7 mm of lateral column is involved, the radial head engages the defect inhibiting marrow-stimulated fibrocartilage repair and possibly leading to accelerated radiocapitellar arthrosis. For these larger engaging defects removal of the loose fragments and osteochondral restoration by means of mosaicplasty or osteochondral autograft transfer system (OATS) is the preferred treatment. In the case of partially detached fragments, the detached portion (usually central) should be debrided from the unstable central area to a stable lateral rim. Once stable osteochondral borders have been obtained, the lesion is carefully examined arthroscopically to determine how much of the lateral column is involved and if the radial head engages with the defect. Chappell and ElAttrache[38] reported that lesions greater than 1 cm^2 (mean 1.32 cm^2) that did not have lateral column involvement were treated successfully with microfracture, whereas those involving the lateral column did well with osteochondral grafting.

Fragment fixation

Fragment fixation has been used to treat unstable, partially detached OCD lesions.[34] Kuwahata and colleagues[35] described open cancellous bone grafting with Herbert screw fixation. At 2.75 years follow-up all patients had returned to sport. Takeda and colleagues[39] reported 10 of 11 male baseball players treated with bone grafting and fragment fixation with radiographically confirmed bony union. Takahara and colleagues[36,37] used an open approach to fix partially detached lesions with lateral olecranon bone pegs. Although these investigators have reported encouraging results, the bone quality on the fragment has limited healing potential. Fragment fixation can be considered, but we have had more consistent results with grafting.

Type III: Chronic Lesions with Loose Bodies

Type III lesions are severe chronic lesions with loose bodies. An acutely displaced OCD can be fixed back to its bed but the healing potential of the fragment may be poor. Osteochondral grafting or drilling may be performed with the same criteria as for type II lesions.

Radial Head Involvement

Athletes typically do not present with combined radial head and capitellar pathology, which has a poor natural history. Our preferred treatment of capitellar OCD depends on the size of the radial head lesion. When lesions are less than 30% of the radial head, treatment should proceed based on the capitellar lesion, as defined earlier.[20] In those patients with severe radiocapitellar degenerative arthritis, mosaicplasty is avoided.

Operative technique

Standard arthroscopic portals are created and the anterior compartment of the elbow is examined. The anterior capitellum is typically normal with most OCD pathology found posteriorly. An arthroscopic valgus stress test may be performed at 70° of flexion while visualizing the ulnohumeral articulation; widening of 2 mm supports an UCL injury. Diagnostic arthroscopy then proceeds in the posterior compartment with standard portals to assess loose bodies and other pathology. OCD fragments are commonly identified in the olecranon fossa and a thorough search for all loose bodies is performed.

Visualization of the capitellum, radial head, trochlear notch, and trochlear ridge can be obtained from a posterolateral portal or direct midlateral portal. A working portal is created in the soft spot or adjacent and slightly ulnar to the established midlateral portal. A cadaver study recently supported use of dual direct lateral portals and documented excellent exposure to the capitellum.[40] Occasionally, patients with OCD and lateral compartment symptoms have a thickened radiocapitellar plica, and if identified, the plica should be resected. The OCD lesion is visualized and graded according to the criteria described earlier. The size and the ability of the capitellum to buttress the radial head is evaluated. At this point, specific procedures are performed as indicated.

Stage 1 lesions with cartilage fibrillation and fissuring are treated with transarticular or retrograde drilling with small 1.14-mm (0.045-in) Kirschner wire. For stage 2 and 3 lesions, detached fragments or loose bodies are removed. Viewing from the postero-lateral or direct lateral portal, a 1.14-mm (0.045-in) or 1.5-mm (0.062-in) Kirschner wire is placed through the accessory lateral portal and vascular channels are created in the lesion separated by 2 mm (**Fig. 7**). A study by Chappell and ElAttrache[38] reported excellent results in 11 patients treated with this indication and technique. The size of the OCD lesions ranged from 7 × 6 mm to 17 × 15 mm.

When mosaicplasty is indicated, small-sized osteochondral autografts are obtained from the knee at the lateral aspect of the femoral condyles above the sulcus terminalis or above the intercondylar notch and transplanted to prepared osteochondral defects on the capitellum.[41] A midlateral working portal is established to debride the lesion to a stable articular rim. In the case of a partially detached fragment, the authors recommend debriding the partially detached portion beginning centrally and proceeding laterally, toward the lateral column. Debridement proceeds until an area of bony integrity is encountered. Osteochondral grafting proceeds if more than 6 to 7 mm of the lateral column is involved or the radial head engages in the defect.

The elbow is flexed to 90° to 100° and a spinal needle is introduced through the anconeus to obtain a perpendicular approach to the lesion. An incision large enough for a 4- to 6-mm-diameter plug is made. The recipient site is drilled perpendicular to the chondral surface using commercially available OATS instrumentation. A donor osteochondral plug is then harvested arthroscopically from the intercondylar notch or lateral edge of the femoral condyle. The donor plug is introduced into the recipient site and impacted flush with the surrounding cartilage (**Fig. 8**). Grafting is repeated as necessary until the lateral column is adequately restored. Drilling can be used if some edges of the lesion cannot be completely replaced. If autograft is undesired, allograft or synthetic scaffolding can be used.

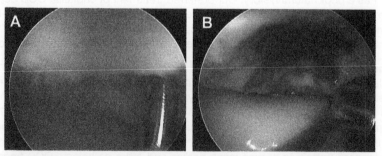

Fig. 7. Microfracture technique. (*A*) A 1.5-mm (0.062-in) Kirschner wire is inserted through the accessory midlateral portal and used to perforate the lesion. (*B*) Bleeding response from the drilling visualized after tourniquet deflated. (*Reproduced from* Ahmad CS, ElAttrache NS. In: Morrey BF, Sanchez-Sotelo J. The elbow and its disorders. 4th edition. Philadelphia: Saunders Elsevier; 2009. p. 591; with permission.)

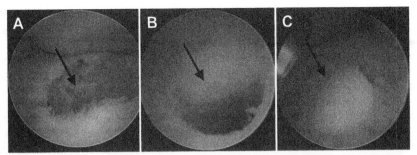

Fig. 8. Osteochondral autograft technique. (*A*) OCD lesion debrided to a stable rim. (*B*) Recipient sight drilled perpendicular to cartilage surface. (*C*) Donor graft in place, flush with cartilage surface. (*Reproduced from* Ahmad CS, ElAttrache NS. Mossicplasty for capitellar OCD. In: Yamaguchi K, American Shoulder and Elbow Surgeons, American Academy of Orthopaedic Surgeons, editors. Advanced reconstruction elbow. 1st edition. Rosemont (IL): American Academy of Orthopaedic Surgeons; 2007. p. 182; with permission.)

Iwasaki and colleagues[41] reported good or excellent results in 7 out of 8 teenaged baseball players with OCD treated with mosaicplasty, 6 returned to competitive baseball. Yamamoto and colleagues[42] reported 6 of 9 young baseball players with grade 3 and 8 of 9 with grade 4 OCD lesions returned to competitive baseball after an OATS procedure. Chappell and ElAttrache[38] also treated 5 baseball players with OCD using an OATS procedure. All 5 returned to competitive baseball and were still playing 5 years postoperatively. The procedure is indicated when more than 6 to 7 mm of the lateral column is involved, and the radial head engages the lesion on careful arthroscopic examination during supination/pronation of the extended arm.

Postoperatively, all patients should be protected for 2 to 3 weeks with a hinged brace. Passive and active assisted motion is performed to avoid postoperative stiffness. Gentle strengthening exercises are initiated at 3 months, progressing to greater strengthening at 4 months. Depending on the sport, a throwing program is initiated at 5 months. Full return to sport can usually be achieved at 6 to 8 months. Rehabilitation is modified for cases of simple debridement and drilling and can return players to sport at 4 or 5 months.

Outcomes

Reports demonstrate long-term follow-up of nonoperative treatment of capitellar OCD has a higher than 50% incidence of impaired motion, pain, and radiographic signs of degenerative joint disease.[43] Several factors influence the overall prognosis. Patient-specific factors include skeletal maturity and type of sport played. Lesion-specific characteristics include size, location, and quality of underlying bone. Early identification and treatment of OCD may improve the long-term poor prognosis. Matsuura and colleagues[44] demonstrated that 91% of cases of early stage OCD responded well to nonoperative treatment, whereas only 50% of cases of advanced stage OCD responded well. Mitsunaga and colleagues[45] noted inferior outcomes in those patients with loose bodies or a delay in surgical treatment. In general, better results are observed when treating younger patients and with open growth plates.[36,37,46,47] Takahara and colleagues[36,37] identified characteristics of an open capitellar growth plate and good elbow motion as better prognosis with nonoperative treatment. However, most cases of OCD are diagnosed as type II lesions and fragment stability affects the final outcome.

Reports vary on return to sports following capitellar OCD. Some studies report that female gymnasts have a particularly low rate of return to sports.[48,49] Jackson and colleagues[48] treated 10 female gymnasts with removal of loose bodies and drilling after failure of nonoperative treatment with only 1 patient returning to sport. However, more recently, Bojanic and colleagues[50] found that 3 of 3 gymnasts successfully returned to their previous level of competition after loose body removal and microfracture. Byrd and colleagues[51] reported 4 of 10 adolescent baseball players were able to return to competitive baseball after osteochondral autografts. However, Yamamoto and colleagues[42] reported 14 of 18 returned after this procedure. McManama and colleagues[52] reported on 14 patients who were treated for OCD of the capitellum and showed that 85% returned to competitive athletics without restrictions at an average follow-up of 2 years. Baumgarten and colleagues[53] reviewed 17 patients who were treated arthroscopically for OCD of the capitellum in the young population. Thirteen of 17 athletes were able to return to sports and were pain free. Chappell and ElAttrache[38] had 8 of 8 male baseball players return to their sport and previous level at an average 3 years follow-up after either microfracture or osteochondral autografting.

Extensor Tendon Enesthopathy/Tennis Elbow

Lateral epicondylitis causes lateral elbow pain in combination with strenuous activity. The patient's pain results from chronic tendinitis of the extensor muscles, in particular the extensor carpi radialis brevis, which is often caused by overuse. Although more common in athletes aged 35 to 50 years, it has also been observed in pediatric tennis players.[54] Prevention strategies include warming up before exercise, good technique, avoiding overtraining, and proper conditioning. Risk factors for prolonged symptoms lasting greater than 6 months include heavier and stiffer racquets, incorrect grip size, inexperience, and poor backhand technique.[55] Pain is reproduced with active wrist extension or passive wrist flexion. Tenderness is localized 1 to 2 cm distal to the lateral epicondyle. Pain may also be elicited at the same area of tenderness by grasping with the fingers while the wrist is kept in extension. Radiographs are typically normal.

Treatment involves avoidance of painful activities, ice, nonsteroidal antiinflammatory drugs (NSAIDs), tennis elbow bracing, racquet modifications, and training modifications.[49] Corticosteroid injections are generally not recommended and necessary in pediatric patients. Operative management in the form of drilling of the lateral epicondyle to stimulate healing may be considered if the patient's pain does not resolve with a year of nonoperative management.[54]

Radiocapitellar Plica

Lateral elbow pain can be also be caused by a thickened radiocapitellar plica alone or in combination with capitellar OCD.[56–58] Patients report lateral sided painful clicking or catching and effusions. The flexion-pronation test may reproduce the click and pain and is performed by passively moving the patients extended elbow into flexion with the forearm pronated. Patients with suspected isolated synovial plica are initially treated with rest and antiinflammatory medication. After 3–6 months of unsuccessful nonoperative treatment, arthroscopic debridement is indicated. Whereas/although no studies are dedicated to youth athletes with radiocapitellar plica, several reports in adults report excellent results with arthroscopic treatment. Kim and colleagues[57] reported excellent results in 11 of 12 patients after debridement of a synovial plica in throwing athletes and golfers. Antuna and O'Driscoll reported on 14 patients with radiocapitellar plica who had painful elbow snapping. Twelve patients had complete relief of their symptoms after resection.[56] Ruch and colleagues[59] demonstrated that radiocapitellar plica may be the cause of vague lateral elbow pain. Eight of the ten patients had good outcomes following surgery.

The camera is introduced in the proximal anteromedial portal and a proximal anterolateral working portal is established. Debridement of synovitis around the radial head is performed. The lateral plica is visualized as a thick fibrous band that snaps back more than the radial neck and head during elbow flexion and extension (**Fig. 9**). An area of chondomalacia is commonly visualized on the anterolateral radial head. Arthroscopic baskets and shavers are used to resect the plica back to the normal annular ligament. The arthroscope is then placed in the posterolateral portal or direct midlateral portal and the plica excision is continued from the midlateral portal (if visualizing from posterolateral portal) or from an accessory midlateral portal (if visualizing from midlateral portal).

POSTERIOR ELBOW INJURIES
Olecranon Apophyseal Injury/Olecranon Stress Fracture

The proximal ulnar ossification center forms at age 8 in girls and age 10 in boys, and closure usually occurs about 6 years later.[60] During the acceleration phase of throwing, or tumbling exercises in gymnastics, the triceps forcefully contracts, and in children with open physes, the force is directly perpendicular to the olecranon apophysis. Because the physis is biomechanically weaker than bone, these repetitive powerful contractions can cause injury to the apophysis. The apophysis widens and fails to close. In patients with a closed olecranon apophysis, a stress fracture may result from the same pathomechanics of repetitive abutment of the olecranon into the olecranon fossa combined with valgus torques, resulting in impaction and shear along the posteromedial olecranon. Thus children develop apophysitis, adolescents develop avulsion fracture, and adults develop posteromedial osteophytes or olecranon stress fracture.

Patients complain of pain, weakness, decreased range of motion and posterior elbow swelling. Pain is specifically located on the bone of the olecranon. Pain that is located more proximally, or with associated snapping would suggest tendonitis or snapping triceps, but this is rare in the younger population. Pain more than the posteromedial ulna in patients with closed olecranon apophyses should raise concern for

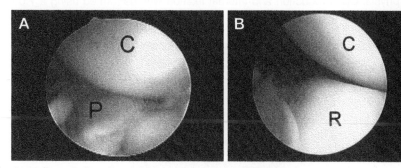

Fig. 9. Radiocapitellar plica. (*A*) Radiocapitellar plica (P) adjacent to capitellum (C). (*B*) After plica excision of radial head (R) and capitellum (C) articulation is unobstructed. (*Reproduced from* Ahmad CS. In: Galatz LM, American Shoulder and Elbow Surgeon, American Academy of Orthopaedic Surgeons, editors. Orthopaedic knowledge update. Shoulder and elbow 3. 3rd edition. Rosemont (IL): American Academy of Orthopaedic Surgeons; 2008. p. 457 and Fig. 10A; with permission.)

olecranon stress fracture, or posteromedial impingement. Throwers have pain during follow-through. Physical examination reveals mild swelling and tenderness to palpation more than the proximal ulna and resisted elbow extension reproduces pain. The extension impingement test is performed by snapping the flexed elbow into full extension causing the olecranon to be driven into the olecranon fossa which reproduces symptoms. The arm bar test is performed with the patient's shoulder in 90° of forward elevation and full internal rotation. The patient's hand is placed on the examiner's shoulder, the examiner places a downward force on the olecranon, levering the elbow that is in full extension (**Fig. 10**).[61] The extension impingement test and arm bar test accurately identify posteromedial impingement in the adult population and most olecranon based pain in the younger population.

Radiographs classically show widening, fragmentation and periphyseal sclerosis, but may be normal. Contralateral radiographs should be obtained for comparison. An MRI or bone scan may be used to confirm the diagnosis of physeal injury, or stress fracture.[2] MRI will typically show enhancement on the T2 sequence.[62] CT scan can also be useful to better evaluate the orientation of the fracture and degree of sclerosis.

Initial treatment of olecranon apophysitis and olecranon stress fractures consist of activity modification, NSAIDs, ice and physical therapy. If symptoms persist, surgical treatment is indicated. In patients with a persistent olecranon physis, radiographic classification may be useful in when determining a treatment plan. Matsuura and colleagues[44] found that absence of periphyseal sclerosis had a high percentage of healing whereas those athletes with sclerosis failed non-operative treatment. Schickendantz and colleagues[62] evaluated 7 professional baseball players with documented olecranon stress fracture and found that all 7 healed with nonoperative treatment.

Surgical treatment is indicated in persistent olecranon physis or olecranon stress fractures, when 3–6 months of non-operative treatment management fails. In patients radiographic sclerosis, early surgery may be indicated. Internal fixation has reported good results. Rudzki and colleagues[63] recommended a single cancellous bone screw, whereas/although others recommend tension band wiring.[44] Charlton and Chandler reviewed 5 maturing adolescent baseball players with pain associated with persistence of the olecranon physis. At an average follow-up of 32 months, all 5 were satisfied with their results. All players returned to their previous level of competition after stabilization with internal fixation and bone grafting. Rettig and colleagues[64] described 5 adolescent baseball pitchers who were diagnosed with persistent olecranon physis. Open reduction and internal fixation was performed using a 7.0 mm

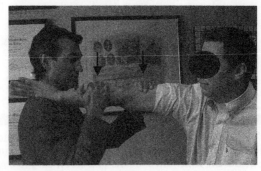

Fig. 10. The arm bar test. The wrist is rested on the examiners shoulder and the patients elbow is levered while in full extension. (*Courtesy of* Center for Shoulder, Elbow and Sports Medicine at Columbia University.)

cancellous screw and washer. One patient had a delayed union, but all patients returned to their previous levels of activities at an average of 30 weeks. Postoperatively, patients are immobilized for 10 days, and active extension is prohibited for 6 weeks. At 8 weeks, active strengthening is implemented. Return to sports is usually allowed at 3 months if clinically asymptomatic. **Fig. 11** is an example of persistent olecranon physis that required screw fixation to go on to full healing.

MEDIAL ELBOW INJURIES

Medial-sided elbow injuries can be either be acute or chronic. For instance a history of pitching would predispose a patient to a chronic overuse injury mechanism. In pitchers valgus extension overload, known as Little Leaguer's elbow, causes a tensile stress on the medial elbow. This medial tensile stress may lead to a spectrum of associated conditions including medial epicondylar aphophysitis, medial epicondylar avulsions, sublime tubercle fractures, UCL sprains and tears, and common wrist flexor and pronator strains.

The pathology associated with medial elbow injuries is strongly influenced by skeletal maturity particularly because the medial epicondyle is the last physis to close. The physis is weaker than the UCL, explaining the higher rate of medial epicondylar avulsions compared with UCL tears in skeletally immature patients. In young patients with throwing related elbow injuries, comparison of radiographs from both elbows may demonstrate broadening of the physeal line of the affected elbow.[65] Consequently knowledge of the mechanisms of injury specific to pediatric patients, medial tensile stress and an open medial epicondyle physis, will allow proper treatment of medial-sided elbow injury.

Medial Epicondylar Apophysitis (Little League Elbow)

Although often applied to any condition that causes pain in a young thrower, Little League elbow most accurately describes medial epicondylar apophysitis.[12] Medial epicondylar apophysitis is a traction injury to the medial epicondylar apophysis most often related to throwing. In individuals approaching skeletal maturity, the medial

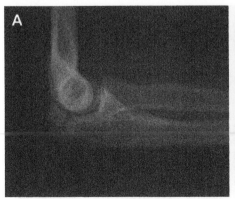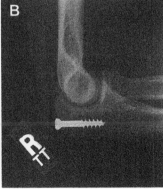

Fig. 11. Persistent olecranon physis. (*A*) Persistent olecranon physis. Note periphyseal sclerosis. (*B*) Screw fixation of persistent olecranon physis that went on to full healing. (*Reproduced from* ElAttrache NS, Ahmad CS. Valgus extension overload and olecranon stress fractures. Sports Med Arthrosc Rev 2003;11:25–9; with permission.)

epicondyle apophysis may fail to close. In more mature athletes, the apophysis may close and injury may occur in the UCL substance or attachment sites.[66]

Patients typically have pain during late cocking and early acceleration when valgus loads are maximal, and when eccentric contraction of the FDS and FCU to stabilize the elbow. Physical examination demonstrates tenderness and swelling more than the medial epicondyle. Occasionally, a mild loss of elbow range of motion is present. There is typically no evidence of valgus instability. Radiographs may reveal widening or fragmentation of the epicondyle ossification center (**Fig. 12**). With chronicity, accelerated growth and gradual deformity of the epicondyle can be seen. In patients nearing skeletally maturity, radiographs may demonstrate a persistent open medial epicondyle apophysis. In addition, changes in the radiocapitellar joint may signal long standing pathology with compression overload laterally.

Management of medial epicondyle apophysitis includes cessation of pitching activities for 4–6 weeks. In the early stages of recovery, ice, and NSAIDs can be useful. If patients present with a flexion contracture, an elbow extension brace can be beneficial. Other strength and conditioning activities should be performed. Occasionally, symptoms return, usually from an inadequate recovery period. In these cases, a splint may be used to more definitively rest the elbow. After the 4- to 6-week rest period, when symptoms have abated, a progressive throwing program is instituted over a 4- to 8-week period. Players typically return to full effort throwing by 12 weeks. Pitchers may elect a position change such as first base, which allows continued participation but with decreased stress to the elbow to avoid recurrence in the same season. If symptoms recur after a trial of nonoperative treatment, then cessation of play for a complete season is indicated.

Medial Epicondyle Avulsion

Avulsion of the medial epicondyle may occur from acute trauma or from repetitive valgus forces. Whereas in childhood, valgus stress overload usually causes microtrauma to the apophysis, in adolescence it more frequently leads to partial or complete medial epicondyle avulsion fractures.[67] In children, medial epicondyle avulsion occurs most commonly in the setting of an elbow dislocation.[68] On physical examination, the patient has loss of motion and exquisite tenderness in the medial

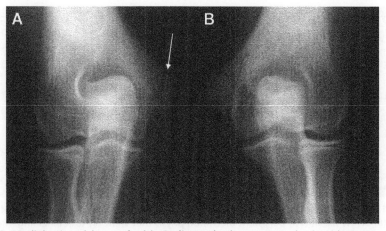

Fig. 12. Medial epicondyle apophysitis. Radiographs demonstrate classic widening and sclerosis of the medial apophyseal ossification center.

epicondyle. The amount of displacement of the bone fragment is dependent on the soft tissue attachments. Woods and Tullos[69] classified medial epicondyle avulsions into 2 categories. Type I fractures occur in young children and are caused by the pull of the anterior band of the UCL. A large and rotated fragment is produced. In adolescent patients, an avulsion fracture caused by a flexor tendon attachment leaves the ligamentous attachments intact. This typically results in a smaller fracture fragment and is categorized as a type II fracture.

Although the decision between nonoperative and operative treatment remains controversial, the main criteria consists of displacement, fracture stability, and age. Conservative treatment with splint immobilization for 5 to 7 days, followed by early range of motion should be instituted for fractures with less than 5 mm displacement. However, a retrospective study by Farsetti and colleagues[70] demonstrated that nonsurgical and surgical treatments of medial epicondyle fractures with 5- to 15-mm displacement had comparable results at a mean follow-up of 34 years. Other studies have also suggested that nonunion or fracture displacement does not influence outcome.[71–73]

Nevertheless some investigators suggest that open reduction and internal fixation may be considered for athletes who throw especially when instability is identified or greater than 5-mm displacement exists.[69,74,75] Good results are reported with operative treatment.[74] A stress test radiograph may be performed to assess valgus instability. In young children, smooth pins are used to preserve the apophysis. With adolescents with large fragments, screw fixation is preferred. For small comminuted fragments with instability and a positive stress test, fragment excision and reattachment of the ligamentous complex is indicated. **Fig. 13** shows screw fixation for a displaced apophyseal fracture.

Sublime Tubercle Avulsion

Avulsion of the sublime tubercle has been reported in young throwers. In 1 study, the average age at the time of injury was 16.9 years. Players commonly present with acute

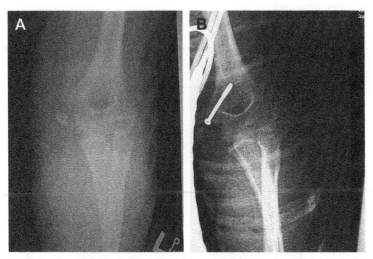

Fig. 13. Medial epicondylar apophyseal avulsion. (*A*) Displaced medial epicondylar apophyseal avulsion fracture. (*B*) Screw fixation for displaced medial epicondylar apophyseal avulsion fracture. (*Courtesy of* Center for Shoulder, Elbow and Sports Medicine at Columbia University.)

pain over the proximal medial ulna associated with throwing. Radiographs confirm a small fleck of bone off the sublime tubercle (**Fig. 14**), and MRI sequences may confirm the small piece of bone attached to the sublime tubercle.

Treatment includes a period of immobilization in a brace locked at 90° for 1 week. Then passive range-of-motion exercises are allowed in the brace for 6 weeks. At 8 weeks, a progressive throwing program is instituted, and by 12 weeks, all players can resume competitive throwing. Salvo and colleagues[76] recommended fixation with suture anchors when nonoperative treatment failed. If fixation was inadequate in the avulsed tubercle, a ligament reconstruction was performed with autologous tissue. Postoperatively, the elbow was immobilized in 90° of flexion in a posterior splint for 1 week. Then, the arm was placed in a hinged elbow brace for 3 weeks at 90°. At 3 weeks, active and passive elbow range of motion was allowed. A throwing program was started at 12 weeks and patients were allowed to return to competitive throwing by 6 months. If a formal reconstruction had to be performed, a throwing program was allowed at 6 months, and patients were able to return to competitive throwing at 1 year. All patients returned to their previous level of activity in their series.

Medial Collateral Ligament Injury

Although UCL injuries are believed to be rare among the pediatric population, youth UCL injuries are increasingly being recognized and surgically managed. In children, the injury develops more acutely than in adults. Most patients report a popping sensation, and subsequent swelling and ecchymosis. After an injury, patients who attempt to throw report an inability to compete at their preinjury level. Patients describe pain during late cocking and early acceleration with reduced throwing velocity and control.

Physical examination reveals tenderness over the UCL. The moving valgus stress test described by O'Driscoll and colleagues[77] is performed with the patient in an upright position with the shoulder in 90° of abduction. With the elbow maximally flexed, the examiner applies a valgus stress about the elbow, until the shoulder reaches maximal external rotation. At this time, the elbow is quickly extended to approximately 30°. A positive examination reproduces pain, instability, or apprehension during this maneuver.

The lack of pain with resisted wrist flexion rules out a medial epicondyle avulsion/ medial epicondyle apophysitis or flexor-pronator injury, but both injuries may occur simultaneously. Athletes with UCL injuries commonly present with ulnar neuritis.

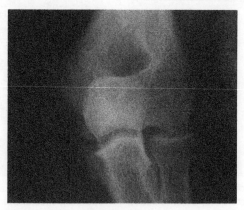

Fig. 14. Avulsion fracture of sublime tubercle. (*Courtesy of* Center for Shoulder, Elbow and Sports Medicine at Columbia University.)

Hand clumsiness or tingling in the ring and small fingers should prompt careful evaluation of the ulnar nerve. When considering surgery, it is important to recognize that up to 30% of patients do not have a palmaris longus tendon.[78]

Plain radiographs infrequently reveal the characteristic findings of UCL injuries, as they do in adult athletes. MRI is the most helpful diagnostic tool, and MRI arthrography is 97% sensitive in detecting UCL injury (**Fig. 15**).[79] In the pediatric population, MRI is also helpful in diagnosing other lesions that may be present including elbow OCD, olecranon physeal injury, or stress reaction.

The management of UCL injuries in the youth athletes involves rest, bracing, NSAIDs, and physical therapy for 6 weeks with a gradual return to activity. Attention must be paid to core, hip, and lower extremity strengthening, in addition to the upper extremity. Motion deficits in the hip and shoulder should be sought and corrected. Proper pitching mechanics and pitching volume guidelines should be recommended. Rettig and colleagues[80] demonstrated a 42% return to same level of play with an average return at 24.5 weeks with nonoperative treatment. No history or physical examination features are predictive for athletes who respond to nonoperative treatment. Local steroid injections should be avoided because they may risk further injury to the UCL.

If conservative treatment fails, the athlete has options to change sport or change position. Patients who wish to continue throwing, have failed nonoperative treatment, have an accurate diagnosis of UCL injury, and are willing to participate in lengthy rehabilitation are indicated for surgical reconstruction. The UCL can be repaired using standard adult techniques or primary repair.[63,81] Savoie and colleagues[82] recently reported on 60 young athletes who underwent primary repair of UCL tears. Good to excellent results were found in 93%, and all but 2 patients returned to the same or higher level of competition. There were 4 failures noted, 2 early and 2 late. The

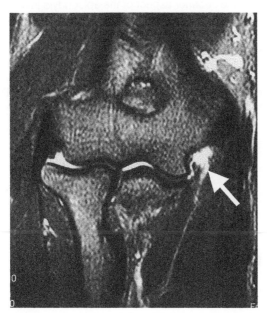

Fig. 15. MRI demonstrating an avulsion of the MCL from its humeral attachment. (*Reproduced from* Rahman RK, Levine WN, Ahmad CS. Curr Rev Musculoskeletal Med 2008;1:200; with permission.)

investigators concluded that primary repair of a proximal or distal ligament injury is a viable option in the young nonprofessional athlete. Postoperatively rehabilitation includes elbow immobilization 1 week in 30° of flexion. Wrist, elbow, and shoulder motion may begin after 1 week. At 4 to 6 weeks, full range of motion should be achieved and active strengthening can begin. At 8 weeks, plyometrics are introduced, and by 6 months, the patient may begin a throwing program. Athletes are allowed to resume competitive throwing by 9 to 12 months.

Several modifications have been made to Frank W. Jobe's original description of UCL reconstruction. A skin incision is centered over the medial epicondyle. The sensory branches of the medial antebrachial cutaneous nerve are protected. The flexor-pronator mass is split exposing the medial collateral ligament (MCL). A longitudinal split is made in the ligament and valgus stress reveals opening of the ulnohumeral articulation if the MCL is insufficient. Converging 3.2-mm drill holes are made in the ulna at the sublime tubercle. A 4.5-mm inferior drill hole is then made at the site of the anatomic origin of the anterior bundle of MCL on the medial epicondyle that does not penetrate the posterior cortex. Two superior drill holes are placed in the anterosuperior surface of the epicondyle approximately separated by 1 cm and connect to the inferior drill hole. The palmaris longus from the ipsilateral arm is harvested through a series of small transverse incisions. The graft is passed through the proximal ulnar bone tunnel and medial epicondyle in a figure-of-eight configuration and tensioned. Fixation of the graft is achieved with sutures. The native ligament is then repaired over the graft with simple sutures placed.

The docking technique is a modification of the Jobe technique that simplifies graft passage, tensioning, and fixation by using sutures to control to graft limbs passed through the humerus. The docking technique modification uses the muscle splitting approach with tunnel creation on the ulna similar to the Jobe technique. The inferior humeral tunnel position is also similar to the Jobe technique. Two small 2.0-mm exit tunnels are created on the superior aspect of the epicondyle instead of large tunnels. The graft is fashioned to an exact length to fit inside the humeral tunnel. The free ends of the graft are controlled with sutures that are passed through the 2 exit tunnels and tied over a bony bridge (**Fig. 16**).

A new technique of MCL reconstruction achieves ulnar-sided fixation in a single bone tunnel with an interference screw and humeral fixation using the docking technique.[83] This technique is less technically demanding because the number of drill holes required is reduced. This reduces the chance for surgical error. Less dissection

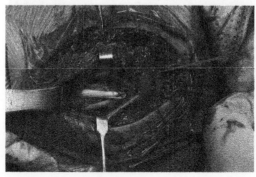

Fig. 16. Sutures are used to tension graft in humeral bone tunnels. (*From* Ahmad CS, ElAttrache NS. Elbow valgus instability in the throwing athlete. J Am Acad Orthop Surg 2006;14 (12):697; with permission.)

through a muscle splitting approach is afforded because only a single central tunnel is required rather than 2 tunnels with an intervening bony bridge on the ulna. Less dissection reduces the amount of inflammation secondary to surgical trauma. With a single tunnel, the posterior ulnar tunnel that is in closest proximity to the ulnar nerve is avoided. Graft passage is less difficult with an interference screw, which is a screw placed between the bone and the graft to afford strong fixation, in a single tunnel. Some surgeons favor screw fixation on the ulna and docking fixation on the humeral epicondyle.[84]

Rehabilitation consists of immediate postoperative elbow immobilization in a splint for 10 days. Then active wrist, elbow, and shoulder range-of-motion exercises are initiated. After 4 to 6 weeks, strengthening exercises are initiated. At 4 months the patient begins a progressive throwing program initially with ball tosses of 9 to 12 m (30 to 40 ft). At 8 to 9 months, pitchers throw from the pitching mound and progress to 70% of maximum effort. Throwing in competition is permitted at 1 year if the shoulder, elbow, and forearm are pain free while throwing and full strength and range of motion have returned. Throughout the rehabilitation phase, careful supervision and focus on body and throwing mechanics should be emphasized.

Petty and colleagues[85] reported on 27 adolescent throwers who required UCL reconstruction. At an average follow-up of 35 months, 74% had returned to baseball at the same or higher level. The investigators concluded that surgical indications for UCL reconstruction in the high school baseball player were different from those in the collegiate or professional player. The decision to proceed with surgery is more complex in this age group because their current level of competition and future potential may not warrant surgery. In addition, the results of surgery were inferior to results in older mature athletes.

INJURY PREVENTION

Prevention of elbow injury is paramount to slow the current trend of increasing elbow injuries in our youth athletes. Inappropriate throwing volume is the most biggest risk for elbow injuries. Young athletes now participate in year-round baseball, play for a multiple teams, participate in camps, clinics, and intensive showcases.[86] Olsen and colleagues[86] reported that pitching more than 8 months a year and pitching more than 80 pitches per game increased the risk for elbow surgery 5-fold and 4-fold, respectively. Other studies have demonstrated that elbow pain is associated with duration of annual play, number of pitches, arm fatigue, increased age and weight, and weight lifting.[25,86,87] Throwers often participate in off-season weight training programs for other sports such as football.

Pitch type also influences the risk of elbow injury.[25,87] Different pitches can influence torque production on the elbow, although there is no definite consensus on which pitch is the most dangerous. The mechanical differences of pitch type have demonstrated similar motions for the fastball and slider, but the curveball has more forearm supination, less wrist extension, and a shorter stride and slower trunk rotation than both the fastball and change-up.[88] In adult pitchers, Escamilla and colleagues[89] showed that the fastball and slider produced the highest forces on the shoulder and elbow. Fleisig and colleagues[90] found instead that the curveball generated the highest elbow valgus stress in collegiate pitchers. The change-up was safer than either the curveball or the fastball. In children, Lyman and colleagues[25] concluded that the splitter and slider increased the odds for elbow pain in pitchers aged 9 to 12 years.[87] There is evidence to suggest that a curveball is associated with a 52% increased risk of shoulder pain and a slider is associated with an 85% increased risk of elbow pain.[87]

Although there is no consensus, the studies suggest that pitches other than the change-up exert significant torque on the elbow. Because the better Little League players tend to be the ones that pitch fastballs and curveballs, they may be at risk for injury, especially because these better players generally pitch more often and on more teams.

Improper throwing mechanics are common in the injured athletes. Most mechanical issues are caused by poor execution, poor coaching, and physical limitations. Many young athletes are coached by parents who may be less knowledgeable of proper throwing mechanics and injuries compared with trained pitching coaches. Participation on multiple teams also leads to varied and conflicting instruction. Poor mechanics typically leads to early fatigue, breakdown, and injury especially in conjunction with excessive volume. Frequently, improper arm mechanics are initiated by poor use of the lower extremities. Poor stride and foot placement typically leads to compensations further up the kinetic chain, and alterations in arm angle can lead to increased stress on the pitching arm. For example, a flattened arm angle is routinely the result of a closed foot placement of the plant foot resulting in the athlete throwing across the body. This leads to increased valgus stress on the elbow. It may also lead to decreased velocity, which forces the athlete to increase their effort further, increasing the abnormal stress on the arm. Both of these scenarios can often be traced to poor strength or flexibility of the lower extremities, so it is imperative that the evaluation of the young thrower with upper extremity symptoms also includes the lower extremities and trunk.

The USA Baseball Medical and Safety Advisory Committee has created guidelines that have been reviewed and recently updated.[87,91] The most recent Committee report (May 2006) advocates that children learn pitches according to the following: fastball at age 8 years; change-up at age 10 years; curveball at age 14 years; knuckleball at age 15 years; slider/forkball/splitter/screwball at more than age 16 years. Maximum pitch counts per game are given according to age. In addition, pitching is limited to 9 months per year and all overhead activities should be avoided during those 3 months of rest. During the season, a pitcher should be removed immediately if pain is felt with throwing, should never return to the pitch the same day after being removed, and should not practice competitive pitches after the game. Pitchers less than 13 years old should have at least 3 days rest after throwing more than 4 innings. Pitchers aged 13 to 18 years require at least 3 days rest after throwing more than 5 innings. Often overlooked but pitchers should not play as a catcher when not pitching.

SUMMARY

Elbow injuries in the pediatric and adolescent population represent a spectrum of pathology that can be categorized as medial tension injuries, lateral compression injuries, and posterior shear injuries. Early and accurate diagnosis can improve outcomes of nonoperative and operative treatment. Prevention strategies are important to help reduce the increasing incidence of elbow injuries in youth athletes.

REFERENCES

1. Benjamin HJ, Briner WW Jr. Little League elbow. Clin J Sport Med 2005;15(1):
   37–40.
2. Ireland ML, Hutchinson MR. Upper extremity injuries in young athletes. Clin
   Sports Med 1995;14(3):533–69.
3. Park MC, Ahmad CS. Dynamic contributions of the flexor-pronator mass to elbow
   valgus stability. J Bone Joint Surg Am 2004;86(10):2268–74.

4. Safran M, Ahmad CS, ElAttrache NS. Ulnar collateral ligament of the elbow. Arthroscopy 2005;21(11):1381–95.
5. Cain EL Jr, Dugas JR, Wolf RS, et al. Elbow injuries in throwing athletes: a current concepts review. Am J Sports Med 2003;31(4):621–35.
6. Hamilton CD, Glousman RE, Jobe FW, et al. Dynamic stability of the elbow: electromyographic analysis of the flexor pronator group and the extensor group in pitchers with valgus instability. J Shoulder Elbow Surg 1996;5(5):347–54.
7. Altchek D, Andrews JR. The athlete's elbow. Philadelphia: Lippincott Williams & Wilkins; 2001.
8. DeLee J, Drez D, Stanitski CL. Orthopaedic sports medicine: principles and practice. Philadelphia: WB Saunders; 1994.
9. Fleisig GS, Barrentine SW, Zheng N, et al. Kinematic and kinetic comparison of baseball pitching among various levels of development. J Biomech 1999; 32(12):1371–5.
10. Campbell KR, HS, Takagi Y, et al. Kinetic analysis of the elbow and shoulder in professional and Little League pitchers. Med Sci Sports Exerc 1994; 26(Suppl):S175.
11. Limpisvasti O. Video motion analysis of developing throwers. Paper presented at: AAOS 2008 Annual Meeting. San Francisco (CA), March 3–5, 2008.
12. Barnes DA, Tullos HS. An analysis of 100 symptomatic baseball players. Am J Sports Med 1978;6(2):62–7.
13. Callaway GH, Field LD, Deng XH, et al. Biomechanical evaluation of the medial collateral ligament of the elbow. J Bone Joint Surg Am 1997;79(8): 1223–31.
14. Fleisig GS, Barrentine SW, Escamilla RF, et al. Biomechanics of overhand throwing with implications for injuries. Sports Med 1996;21(6):421–37.
15. Fleisig GS, Andrews JR, Dillman CJ, et al. Kinetics of baseball pitching with implications about injury mechanisms. Am J Sports Med 1995;23(2):233–9.
16. Werner SL, Fleisig GS, Dillman CJ, et al. Biomechanics of the elbow during baseball pitching. J Orthop Sports Phys Ther 1993;17(6):274–8.
17. Ahmad CS, Lee TQ, ElAttrache NS. Biomechanical evaluation of a new ulnar collateral ligament reconstruction technique with interference screw fixation. Am J Sports Med 2003;31(3):332–7.
18. Panner H. An affection of the capitulum humeri resembling Calve-Perthes disease of the hip. Acta Radiol 1927;8:617–8.
19. Laurent LE, Lindstrom BL. Osteochondrosis of the capitellum humeri: Panner's disease. Acta Orthop Scand 1956;26:111–9.
20. Kobayashi K, Burton KJ, Rodner C, et al. Lateral compression injuries in the pediatric elbow: Panner's disease and osteochondritis dissecans of the capitellum. J Am Acad Orthop Surg 2004;12(4):246–54.
21. Voloshin I, Schena A. Elbow injuries. In: Schepsis AA, Busconi BD, editors. Sports medicine, vol. 1. Philadelphia: Lippincott Williams & Wilkins; 2006. p. 285–300.
22. Ruch DS, Poehling GG. Arthroscopic treatment of Panner's disease. Clin Sports Med 1991;10(3):629–36.
23. Singer KM, Roy SP. Osteochondrosis of the humeral capitellum. Am J Sports Med 1984;12(5):351–60.
24. Lord J, Winell JJ. Overuse injuries in pediatric athletes. Curr Opin Pediatr 2004; 16(1):47–50.
25. Lyman S, Fleisig GS, Waterbor JW, et al. Longitudinal study of elbow and shoulder pain in youth baseball pitchers. Med Sci Sports Exerc 2001;33(11): 1803–10.

26. Haraldsson S. On osteochondrosis deformas juvenilis capituli humeri including investigation of intra-osseous vasculature in distal humerus. Acta Orthop Scand Suppl 1959;38:1–232.

27. Fa K, E B, U H. Are bone bruises a possible cause of osteochondritis dissecans of the capitellum? A case report and review of the literature. Arch Orthop Trauma Surg 2005;125(8):545–9.

28. Yang Z, Wang Y, Gilula LA, et al. Microcirculation of the distal humeral epiphyseal cartilage: implications for post-traumatic growth deformities. J Hand Surg Am 1998;23(1):165–72.

29. Difelice GS, Meunier MJ, Paletta GA. Elbow injury in the adolescent athlete. In: Altchek DW, Andrews JR, editors. Athlete's elbow. Philadelphia: Lippincott Williams & Wilkins; 2001. p. 231–48.

30. Takahara M, Ogino T, Sasaki I, et al. Long term outcome of osteochondritis dissecans of the humeral capitellum. Clin Orthop Relat Res 1999;363: 108–15.

31. Rosenberg ZS, Beltran J, Cheung YY. Pseudodefect of the capitellum: potential MR imaging pitfall. Radiology 1994;191(3):821–3.

32. Petrie R, Bradley JP. Osteochondritis dissecans of the humeral capitellum. In: De Lee J, Drez D, Miller, editors. Orthopaedic sports medicine: principles and practice. Philadelphia: WB Saunders; 2003. p. 1284–93.

33. Ruch DS, Cory JW, Poehling GG. The arthroscopic management of osteochondritis dissecans of the adolescent elbow. Arthroscopy 1998;14(8):797–803.

34. Larsen MW, Pietrzak WS, DeLee JC. Fixation of osteochondritis dissecans lesions using poly (l-lactic acid)/poly(glycolic acid) copolymer bioabsorbable screws. Am J Sports Med 2005;33(1):68–76.

35. Kuwahata Y, Inoue G. Osteochondritis dissecans of the elbow managed by Herbert screw fixation. Orthopedics 1998;21(4):449–51.

36. Takahara M, Mura N, Sasaki J, et al. Classification, treatment, and outcome of osteochondritis dissecans of the humeral capitellum. J Bone Joint Surg Am 2007;89(6):1205–14.

37. Takahara M, Mura N, Sasaki J, et al. Classification, treatment, and outcome of osteochondritis dissecans of the humeral capitellum. Surgical technique. J Bone Joint Surg Am 2008;90(Suppl 2 Pt 1):47–62.

38. Chappell JD, ElAttrache NS. Clinical outcome of arthroscopic treatment of OCD lesions of the capitellum. Paper presented at: American Orthopaedic Society for Sports Medicine. Orlando (FL), July 10–13, 2008.

39. Takeda H, Watarai K, Matsushita T, et al. A surgical treatment for unstable osteochondritis dissecans lesions of the humeral capitellum in adolescent baseball players. Am J Sports Med 2002;30(5):713–7.

40. Davis JT, Idjadi JA, Siskosky MJ, et al. Dual direct lateral portals for treatment of osteochondritis dissecans of the capitellum: an anatomic study. Arthroscopy 2007;23(7):723–8.

41. Iwasaki N, Kato H, Ishikawa J, et al. Autologous osteochondral mosaicplasty for capitellar osteochondritis dissecans in teenaged patients. Am J Sports Med 2006;34(8):1233–9.

42. Yamamoto Y, Ishibashi Y, Tsuda E, et al. Osteochondral autograft transplantation for osteochondritis dissecans of the elbow in juvenile baseball players: minimum 2-year follow-up. Am J Sports Med 2006;34(5):714–20.

43. Bauer M, Jonsson K, Josefsson PO, et al. Osteochondritis dissecans of the elbow. A long-term follow-up study. Clin Orthop Relat Res 1992;284: 156–60.

44. Matsuura T, Kashiwaguchi S, Iwase T, et al. The value of using radiographic criteria for the treatment of persistent symptomatic olecranon physis in adolescent throwing athletes. Am J Sports Med 2009;38:141–5.

45. Mitsunaga MM, Adishian DA, Bianco AJ Jr. Osteochondritis dissecans of the capitellum. J Trauma 1982;22(1):53–5.

46. Pappas AM. Osteochondrosis dissecans. Clin Orthop Relat Res 1981;158:59–69.

47. Mihara K, Tsutsui H, Nishinaka N, et al. Nonoperative treatment for osteochondritis dissecans of the capitellum. Am J Sports Med 2009;37(2):298–304.

48. Jackson DW, Silvino N, Reiman P. Osteochondritis in the female gymnast's elbow. Arthroscopy 1989;5(2):129–36.

49. Bylak J, Hutchinson MR. Common sports injuries in young tennis players. Sports Med 1998;26(2):119–32.

50. Bojanic I, Ivkovic A, Boric I. Arthroscopy and microfracture technique in the treatment of osteochondritis dissecans of the humeral capitellum: report of three adolescent gymnasts. Knee Surg Sports Traumatol Arthrosc 2006;14(5):491–6.

51. Byrd JW, Jones KS. Arthroscopic surgery for isolated capitellar osteochondritis dissecans in adolescent baseball players: minimum three-year follow-up. Am J Sports Med 2002;30(4):474–8.

52. McManama GB Jr, Micheli LJ, Berry MV, et al. The surgical treatment of osteochondritis of the capitellum. Am J Sports Med 1985;13(1):11–21.

53. Baumgarten TE, Andrews JR, Satterwhite YE. The arthroscopic classification and treatment of osteochondritis dissecans of the capitellum. Am J Sports Med 1998;26(4):520–3.

54. Gregg JR, Torg E. Upper extremity injuries in adolescent tennis players. Clin Sports Med 1988;7(2):371–85.

55. Scuderi GR, McCann PD. Sports medicine: a comprehensive approach. 2nd edition. Philadelphia: Elsevier Mosby; 2005.

56. Antuna SA, O'Driscoll SW. Snapping plicae associated with radiocapitellar chondromalacia. Arthroscopy 2001;17(5):491–5.

57. Kim DH, Gambardella RA, Elattrache NS, et al. Arthroscopic treatment of posterolateral elbow impingement from lateral synovial plicae in throwing athletes and golfers. Am J Sports Med 2006;34(3):438–44.

58. Steinert AF, Goebel S, Rucker A, et al. Snapping elbow caused by hypertrophic synovial plica in the radiohumeral joint: a report of three cases and review of literature. Arch Orthop Trauma Surg 2010;130:347–51.

59. Ruch DS, Papadonikolakis A, Campolattaro RM. The posterolateral plica: a cause of refractory lateral elbow pain. J Shoulder Elbow Surg 2006;15(3):367–70.

60. Flecker H. Time of appearance and fusion of ossification centers as observed by roentgenographic methods. AJR Am J Roentgenol 1942;47:97–159.

61. O'Driscoll S. Valgus extension overload and the symptomatic plica. In: Levine WN, editor. AAOS monograph series: the athlete's elbow. Rosemont (IL): American Academy of Orthopaedic Surgeons; 2008. p. 80–93.

62. Schickendantz MS, Ho CP, Koh J. Stress injury of the proximal ulna in professional baseball players. Am J Sports Med 2002;30(5):737–41.

63. Rudzki JR, Paletta GA Jr. Juvenile and adolescent elbow injuries in sports. Clin Sports Med 2004;23(4):581–608, ix.

64. Rettig AC, Wurth TR, Mieling P. Nonunion of olecranon stress fractures in adolescent baseball pitchers: a case series of 5 athletes. Am J Sports Med 2006;34(4):653–6.

65. Crowther M. Elbow pain in pediatrics. Curr Rev Musculoskelet Med 2009;2(2):83–7.

66. Bradley J, Dandy DJ. Results of drilling osteochondritis dissecans before skeletal maturity. J Bone Joint Surg Br 1989;71(4):642–4.

67. Klingele KE, Kocher MS. Little league elbow: valgus overload injury in the paediatric athlete. Sports Med 2002;32(15):1005–15.

68. Chambers HG. Fractures involving the medial epicondylar apophysis. In: Rockwood CA Jr, Wilkins KE, Beaty JH, editors. Fractures in children. Philadelphia: JB Lippincott; 1996. p. 801–19.

69. Woods GW, Tullos HS. Elbow instability and medial epicondyle fractures. Am J Sports Med 1977;5(1):23–30.

70. Farsetti P, Potenza V, Caterini R, et al. Long-term results of treatment of fractures of the medial humeral epicondyle in children. J Bone Joint Surg Am 2001;83(9): 1299–305.

71. Josefsson PO, Danielsson LG. Epicondylar elbow fracture in children. 35-year follow-up of 56 unreduced cases. Acta Orthop Scand 1986;57(4):313–5.

72. Bede WB, Lefebvre AR, Rosman MA. Fractures of the medial humeral epicondyle in children. Can J Surg 1975;18(2):137–42.

73. Fowles JV, Slimane N, Kassab MT. Elbow dislocation with avulsion of the medial humeral epicondyle. J Bone Joint Surg Br 1990;72(1):102–4.

74. Hines RF, Herndon WA, Evans JP. Operative treatment of medial epicondyle fractures in children. Clin Orthop Relat Res 1987;223:170–4.

75. Jobe FW, Stark H, Lombardo SJ. Reconstruction of the ulnar collateral ligament in athletes. J Bone Joint Surg Am 1986;68(8):1158–63.

76. Salvo JP, Rizio L 3rd, Zvijac JE, et al. Avulsion fracture of the ulnar sublime tubercle in overhead throwing athletes. Am J Sports Med 2002;30(3):426–31.

77. O'Driscoll SW, Lawton RL, Smith AM. The "moving valgus stress test" for medial collateral ligament tears of the elbow. Am J Sports Med 2005;33(2):231–9.

78. Thompson NW, Mockford BJ, Cran GW. Absence of the palmaris longus muscle: a population study. Ulster Med J 2001;70(1):22–4.

79. Azar FM, Andrews JR, Wilk KE, et al. Operative treatment of ulnar collateral ligament injuries of the elbow in athletes. Am J Sports Med 2000;28(1):16–23.

80. Rettig AC, Sherrill C, Snead DS, et al. Nonoperative treatment of ulnar collateral ligament injuries in throwing athletes. Am J Sports Med 2001;29(1):15–7.

81. Argo D, Trenhaile SW, Savoie FH 3rd, et al. Operative treatment of ulnar collateral ligament insufficiency of the elbow in female athletes. Am J Sports Med 2006; 34(3):431–7.

82. Savoie FH 3rd, Trenhaile SW, Roberts J, et al. Primary repair of ulnar collateral ligament injuries of the elbow in young athletes: a case series of injuries to the proximal and distal ends of the ligament. Am J Sports Med 2008;36(6): 1066–72.

83. Koh JL, Schafer MF, Keuter G, et al. Ulnar collateral ligament reconstruction in elite throwing athletes. Arthroscopy 2006;22(11):1187–91.

84. Dines JS, ElAttrache NS, Conway W, et al. Clinical outcomes of the Dane TJ technique to address medial ulnar collateral ligament insufficiency of the elbow. Paper presented at: American Orthopaedic Society for Sports Medicine Annual Meeting. Calgary (Canada), July 15, 2007.

85. Petty DH, Andrews JR, Fleisig GS, et al. Unar collateral ligament injuries in high school baseball players. Clinical results and injury risk factors. Am J Sports Med 2004;32(5):1158–64.

86. Olsen SJ II, Fleisig GS, Dun S, et al. Risk factors for shoulder and elbow injuries in adolescent baseball pitchers. Am J Sports Med 2006;34(6):905–12.

87. Lyman S, Fleisig GS, Andrews JR, et al. Effect of pitch type, pitch count and pitching mechanics on risk of elbow and shoulder pain in youth baseball pitchers. Am J Sports Med 2002;30(4):463–8.

88. Barrentine SW, Fleisig GS, Whiteside JA, et al. Biomechanics of windmill softball pitching with implications about injury mechanisms at the shoulder and elbow. J Orthop Sports Phys Ther 1998;28(6):479–95.

89. Escamilla RF, Fleisig GS, Zheng N, et al. Biomechanics of the knee during closed kinetic chain and open kinetic chain exercises. Med Sci Sports Exerc 1998; 30(4):556–69.

90. Fleisig GS, Kingsley DS, Loftice JW, et al. Kinetic comparison among the fastball, curveball, change-up, and slider in collegiate baseball pitchers. Am J Sports Med 2006;34(3):423–30.

91. Andrews J, Fleisig G. How many pitches should I allow my child to throw? USA Baseball News. April, 1996.

Clinical Concepts for Treatment of the Elbow in the Adolescent Overhead Athlete

Todd S. Ellenbecker, DPT, MS, SCS, OCS, CSCS[a,b,c,]*,
Michael Reinold, DPT, SCS, ATC, CSCS[d], Cory O. Nelson, MD[e]

KEYWORDS

• Injury • Elbow • Adolescent • Overhead athlete

Evaluation and treatment of the elbow in the adolescent overhead athlete requires a comprehensive approach. This comprehensive approach includes a complete upper extremity evaluation; review of, and guidance regarding, control and limitation of the repetitive overhead athletic stress exposures; total arm strength rehabilitation approach; and a guided return to overhead sport program. Although it is beyond the scope of this article to completely cover all aspects of the rehabilitation and prevention strategies, this article discusses some of these concepts as they apply to treatment of the adolescent overhead athlete with an elbow injury.

Repetitive overuse to the adolescent elbow is an inherent characteristic of participation in overhead sports. Throwing sports and tennis place repetitive loads to the adolescent elbow that can result in characteristic injury patterns.[1–3] Increased participation in year-round sports, coupled with an increase in sport specialization at younger ages, have been factors cited to explain the frequent finding of upper extremity injuries in adolescent overhead athletes.[3] This article is a review of pertinent literature in baseball and tennis, because a more complete understanding of the demands and characteristic injury pattern in the elbow of the adolescent athlete is an important part of the evaluation and treatment process.

[a] Scottsdale Sports Clinic, Scottsdale, AZ, USA
[b] Exton, PA, USA
[c] ATP World Tour, Scottsdale, Ponte Vedra Beach, FL, USA
[d] Boston Red Sox Baseball Club, Division Of Sports Medicine, Department Of Orthopaedic Surgery, Massachusetts General Hospital, Boston, MA, USA
[e] Sports Medicine & Arthroscopic Surgery, Scottsdale, AZ, USA
* Corresponding author. Scottsdale Sports Clinic, Scottsdale, AZ.
E-mail address: ellenbeckerpt@cox.net

Clin Sports Med 29 (2010) 705–724
doi:10.1016/j.csm.2010.06.006
0278-5919/10/$ – see front matter © 2010 Elsevier Inc. All rights reserved.

BASEBALL

In the last 2 decades, the incidence of elbow injuries in youth baseball has risen sharply. Epidemiologic studies have shown an incidence of elbow pain in up to 58% of youth baseball players.[4–7] Anecdotal experience led to the perception that throwing certain pitches, specifically a curveball, led to a higher incidence of elbow injuries because of the hypothesized increase in stress to the elbow. However, Lyman and colleagues[7] examined the effect of pitch type on the injury risk in youth baseball pitchers and showed no correlation between elbow injury risk and throwing a curveball.

Dun and colleagues[8] recently assessed the biomechanical differences in pitch types in youth baseball pitchers between the ages of 11 and 14 years. The investigators quantified the expected kinematic differences in forearm position but found that the curveball had significantly less elbow varus torque than the fastball. This finding has also been shown in older teenagers and adult pitchers.[9,10] The results of these biomechanical studies are likely produced by the decreased velocity, and thus force, associated with a curveball in comparison with a fastball. Thus, there is conflicting information between the anecdotal experience and biomechanical data regarding the effect of throwing a curveball on injury risk. There are 2 potential reasons why a curveball may show significantly less stress biomechanically but still result in increased elbow injury risk.

First, although kinetic forces were less during the curveball, kinematic analysis showed a significant difference in forearm position while throwing a curveball.[8,10,11] Although this position of forearm supination itself has not been shown to increase valgus stress,[12] the altered position may change the length-tension relationship of the surrounding musculature. In particular, this may decrease the mechanical advantage of the flexor carpi ulnaris and the flexor digitorum superficialis to dynamically stabilize the elbow joint to prevent valgus torque.[13,14]

Second, anecdotally, it seems that youth pitchers who are able to throw a curveball may have greater success than peers without this ability because of the difficulty of hitting this pitch in youth baseball. Pitchers throwing a curveball tend to perform better and throw more often, making them more susceptible to chronic overuse injuries. Thus players throwing curveballs may have a greater incidence of overuse because of the increased repetitions and exposures. Consequently, the effect of overuse on elbow injuries has gained considerable attention in the past several years. Lyman[7] showed a significant correlation between pitches within a game and in the course of a season on elbow injury risk. Pitchers who threw between 600 and 800 pitches in the course of a season (which is not uncommon) had a 234% greater incidence of elbow injury.[7]

In a comparison between the pitching history of youth baseball players who had undergone elbow surgery and healthy pitchers, Olsen and colleagues[15] found that players with a history of elbow surgery had significantly more games per year (30 vs 19), innings per appearance (5.4 vs 4.3), pitches per game (85 vs 66), and pitches per year (2608 vs 1269) than healthy peers. Players who pitched for more than 8 months of the year had a 5 times higher incidence of elbow surgery. Thus, it seems that overuse may be a more important variable in determining elbow injury risk in youth baseball players. These findings have led to the development and enforcement of several pitch count rules and guidelines in both USA Baseball (**Table 1**) and Little League Baseball (**Tables 2** and **3**). Pitching for multiple teams and different leagues throughout the year has also been discouraged. These new rules have been designed in an attempt to prevent overuse and injuries in youth baseball. At this time, it is unknown how successful these rule changes have been, but they represent

Table 1 USA Baseball Medical & Safety Advisory Committee recommendations for pitch limits with youth pitchers				
Age (y)	Pitches/Game	Pitches/wk	Pitches/Season	Pitches/y
9–10	50	75	1000	2000
11–12	75	100	1000	3000
13–14	75	125	1000	3000

a significant advancement in the effort to reduce elbow injuries in youth baseball players. Further refinement and, potentially, greater restrictions may be necessary.

Davis and colleagues[16] showed the relationship between elbow and shoulder injury and throwing mechanics in elite level pitchers. Their study identified 5 key parameters of observation during the pitching motion in adolescent throwers. These parameters included leading with the hips, hand on top position, arm in throwing position, closed shoulder position, and stride foot toward home plate. Each of these parameters was clearly defined and its relationship to shoulder and elbow pain described. Pitchers who had fewer mechanical errors in their throwing motions had lower incidences of shoulder and elbow injury.[16] This study clearly shows the importance of the proper throwing mechanics and describes 5 key areas of analysis that can be applied when evaluating an adolescent throwing athlete.

TENNIS

The tennis serve places valgus extension load on the human elbow similar to the pattern seen during overhead throwing. Repetitive activation of the forearm and wrist musculature during the serve and groundstrokes can lead to injury, especially of the flexor pronator origin at the medial epicondyle.[17] Research has profiled the number of groundstrokes and serves in a typical elite level tennis match.[18] This research has shown the high number of repetitions of the serve and forehand, both of which require kinetic chain activation patterns[19] and inherently are characterized by concentric internal shoulder rotation, forearm pronation, and wrist flexion muscular activation patterns.[20,21] **Fig. 1** shows the valgus extension overload inherent in the tennis serve and throwing motion and its effect on the human elbow.[22,23] **Fig. 2** shows the elbow position during execution of the modern forehand groundstroke in an elite tennis player. Note the position of elbow flexion and supinated forearm position before and during ball contact. This position of the elbow, coupled with aggressive humeral internal rotation, produces a valgus stress to the elbow and is coupled with

Table 2 Little League Baseball youth pitch count regulation	
Age (y)	Pitches/d
17–18	105
13–16	95
11–12	85
9–10	75
7–8	50

Table 3
Little League Baseball youth recommendations for days of rest between outings

Age (y)	Pitches Thrown	Rest Days
17–18	26–50	1
	51–75	2
	76–105	3
<17	21–40	1
	41–60	2
	>60	3

contraction of the forearm pronators and wrist and finger flexors, which originate at the medial epicondyle of the distal humerus. Overload in this region can lead to medial epicondylitis, flexor pronator muscle overload, and growth plate injury from the repetitive stresses in the adolescent elbow in the elite tennis player.[17,24–26]

Recent research completed by the United States Tennis Association (USTA) Sport Science Committee[27] has provided key epidemiologic information regarding the injury and training characteristics of elite junior tennis players. Prior studies by Reese[28] and others[29] have reported shoulder injury rates of 8% to 24% in elite junior tennis players, but did not specifically report the incidence of elbow injury. In the USTA investigation by Kovacs and colleagues,[27] 861 elite level players were studied between the ages of 10 and 17 years. Overall, 41% of players reported at least 1 overuse injury that limited tennis play and competition in the past year. Elbow injuries comprised 3% of the injuries reported among elite junior players. Furthermore, of the 41% of players reporting a musculoskeletal injury, 33% of these players reported a second musculoskeletal injury during that time period.

Additional characteristics of elite junior tennis players included that, in addition to on-court training, 50% used free weights for training, and 58% and 43% of female and male players used medicine balls for upper body weight training, respectively.

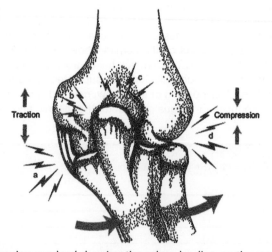

Fig. 1. Valgus extension overload showing the valgus loading on the medial aspect of the elbow and the lateral compression. (*From* Ellenbecker TS, Pieczynski TE, Davies GJ. Rehabilitation of the elbow following sports injury. Clin Sports Med 2010;29:35; with permission.)

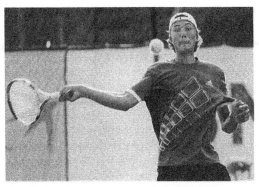

Fig. 2. Modern forehand groundstroke.

Ninety percent of men had a 2-handed backhand, with 97% of women reporting use of a 2-handed backhand. Giangarra and colleagues[30] reported similar patterns of distal upper extremity electromyogram (EMG) activity during a 1- and 2-handed backhand in skilled adult players. Eighty-three percent of the elite juniors report playing predominantly on hard-court surfaces. Present guidelines on number of matches to be played in a year, and the ability to limit the number of serves a player performs, are not as detailed as in baseball. General guidelines from the International Tennis Federation are outlined in **Table 4**.[26] Further research linking tennis play volume and rest intervals are required before more detailed guidelines can be applied in this important area.

SPECIAL CONSIDERATIONS FOR EVALUATION OF THE PEDIATRIC ELBOW

The skeletally immature athlete can present with a variety of complaints in the elbow. A detailed history, physical examination, and radiographic workup are critical in the evaluation. Overuse remains the most common cause of upper extremity pathology in this patient population.[31] The duration and location of the patient's elbow symptoms are important details to elicit from the history. Medial versus lateral pain and acute trauma versus insidious symptoms all aid in directing the physical examination. Skeletal immaturity adds complexity to the evaluation, in that ligamentous and muscular structures commonly injured in adults are generally spared in pediatric patients because the physis is considered the weak link of the elbow structures.

The initial physical examination should include an assessment of the patient's core muscle strength and stability. Simple tests such as single-leg squats or the presence of a Trendelenburg sign can help evaluate the athlete's core. Core weakness and altered throwing mechanics can lead to greater forces being placed on the structures

Table 4
Competitive play recommendations for male elite junior players 15 to 18 years of age (adapted from the International Tennis Federation)[26]

	Player Age (y)	
Variable	15–17	>17
Tournaments/y	18–22	20–30
Matches (singles)	65–80	80–100
Won/loss ratio target	2:1	2:1

of the elbow and potentially increase the risk of injury.[16] Although not within the scope of this article, the importance of a complete examination of both the throwing and nondominant shoulders cannot be understated. Disease states of the elbow may be found in conjunction with shoulder pathology including glenohumeral laxity or instability and rotational motion deficits, which also need to be addressed. A complete neurovascular examination of both extremities is also crucial.

It is helpful for the clinician to examine both elbows in these athletes. The nondominant elbow acts as an internal, normal control, and any asymmetry should alert the examiner to possible pathology. The elbow should be inspected for any obvious swelling or deformity. Acute avulsion fractures may present with ecchymosis. Range of motion of the elbow should be measured both actively and passively. Flexion, extension, supination, and pronation should be evaluated and compared with the nondominant elbow for any side-to-side differences. Generalized ligamentous laxity and elbow hyperextension should be noted because this may be more common in the pediatric population. Acutely injured or inflamed elbows that have an effusion typically demonstrate a loss of extension.

Panner disease and osteochondritis dissecans (OCD) affect the capitellum in this patient population. The radiocapitellar joint should be palpated for crepitation as well as tenderness. Crepitus may be felt in athletes with articular cartilage irregularities in these disease states. A mechanical block to flexion/extension or forearm rotation may be found in patients with loose bodies within the elbow from an unstable OCD lesion.

The medial side of the elbow should be palpated for tenderness at the medial epicondyle, medial ulnar collateral ligament (UCL), and the flexor pronator origin. In skeletally immature patients, the medial epicondyle is more commonly the site of pathology on the medial side of the elbow and should be carefully evaluated. Palpation of the olecranon is also important. Olecranon stress fracture is another injury from overuse more commonly seen in adolescent throwers. Although truly ligamentous injuries in skeletally immature patients are rare, assessing elbow stability remains important. Varus and valgus stability is tested with the elbow held in 25° to 30° of flexion. Acute and displaced medial epicondyle fractures may have significant valgus instability.

RADIOGRAPHS

Standard radiographic evaluation of the elbow includes anteroposterior and lateral views. An oblique or axial flexion view is also commonly ordered. Several adaptive changes, as well as acute injuries, have been described in skeletally immature athletes. The secondary ossification centers of the elbow can vary in formation between sexes and by age, therefore it is helpful to get radiographs of the contralateral elbow and compare any differences (**Fig. 3**). Elbow effusions are most easily seen on the lateral radiograph as a prominence of the posterior fat pad.

Medial Epicondyle

The medial epicondyle is a common site of radiographic findings in Little League baseball players. Hypertrophy of the medial epicondyle or medial humeral cortex, as well as separation and fragmentation of the medial epicondyle, have all been described.[5,31] Separation of the medial epicondyle apophysis has been well documented in this patient population. Hang and colleagues[32] reported a 57% incidence in Little League players. It is thought that these changes are physiologic adaptations to the stresses seen at the medial elbow with repetitive throwing. This must be distinguished from

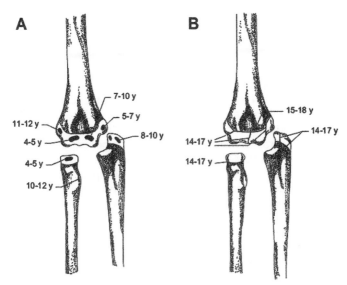

Fig. 3. Growth plates of the human elbow. (*From* Ellenbecker TS, Pieczynski TE, Davies GJ. Rehabilitation of the elbow following sports injury. Clin Sports Med 2010;29:36; with permission.)

an acute medial epicondyle avulsion fracture in which the clinical picture is of an acute injury with sudden pain and swelling usually following a cracking or popping noise in the medial elbow.

Capitellum and Radial Head

High tension forces on the medial aspect of the elbow are usually accompanied by compressive forces seen at the lateral side of the elbow, most commonly involving the capitellum. Panner disease is an articular osteochondrosis usually seen in patients less than 10 years of age, characterized by fissuring, decreased size, and/or fragmentation of the capitellum[33] on plain radiographs. OCD lesions typically are seen as a focal lucency in the subchondral bone of the anterior capitellum. OCD differs from Panner disease in that loose bodies can form from an unstable and detached OCD fragment. Adaptive changes in the radial head can also be seen.

Olecranon

Stress injury occurs at the olecranon from repetitive abutment of the olecranon within the olecranon fossa in extension.[34] Sclerosis within the olecranon can be seen on radiographs with or without a distinct fracture line. Widening of the olecranon epiphysis is seen in the skeletally immature patient.

TOTAL ARM STRENGTH REHABILITATION AND PREVENTION GUIDELINES FOR THE ADOLESCENT OVERHEAD ATHLETE

Rehabilitation and prevention of elbow injuries in the adolescent overhead athlete should include emphasis on the entire upper extremity kinetic chain.[17,19] Inclusion of exercises to address the overall strength and local muscular endurance of the scapular stabilizers, rotator cuff, and distal upper extremity musculature is a critically important part of a successful rehabilitation and prevention program, and is called the total arm strength program.[35]

SCAPULAR STABILIZATION

Kibler[36] has reported extensively on the importance of the scapula in normal upper extremity function in normal function and in overhead sport activities.[37] The primary muscle groups of emphasis are the lower trapezius and serratus anterior force couple.[38] These important muscles work together to provide dynamic stabilization of the scapula. Recent research has confirmed the important of visual observation of the scapula to identify scapular pathology and guide the clinician in the application and progression of resistive exercises to address the scapular dysfunction.[39–42]

For both rehabilitation and prevention of elbow injury, scapular stabilization exercises are emphasized and include external rotation with retraction (**Fig. 4**), an exercise shown to recruit the lower trapezius at a rate 3.3 times more than the upper trapezius, and to use the important position of scapular retraction.[43] Multiple-seated rowing variations are recommended, including the lawn mower exercise (**Fig. 5**) and low-row (**Fig. 6**) variations, which have been studied with EMG quantification by Kibler and colleagues.[44]

Progression to closed-chain exercise using the plus position, which is characterized by maximal scapular protraction, has been recommended by Moseley and colleagues[45] and Decker and colleagues[46] for its inherent maximal serratus anterior recruitment. Closed-chain step-ups (**Fig. 7**), and quadruped position rhythmical stabilization and variations of the pointer position (unilateral arm and ipsilateral leg extension weight bearing) are all used in endurance-oriented formats (timed sets of 30

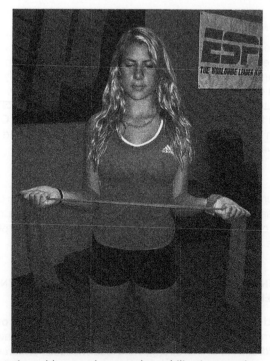

Fig. 4. External rotation with retraction scapular stabilization exercise.

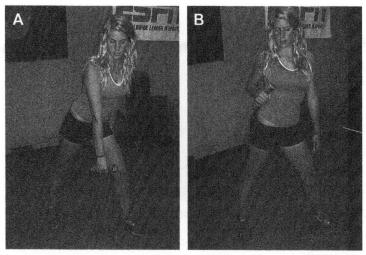

Fig. 5. (*A, B*) Lawnmower scapular stabilization exercise.

seconds or more) to enhance both scapular and trunk stabilization. Push-ups are not recommended because of loading on the anterior aspect of the shoulder during the descent phase of the exercise for overhead throwing athletes. Uhl and colleagues[47] have shown the effects of increasing weight bearing and successive decreases in the number of weight-bearing limbs on muscle activation of the rotator cuff and

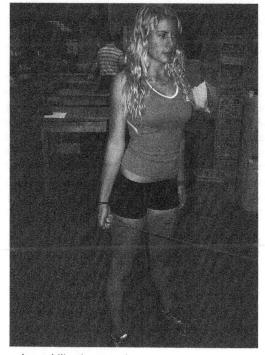

Fig. 6. Low-row scapular stabilization exercise.

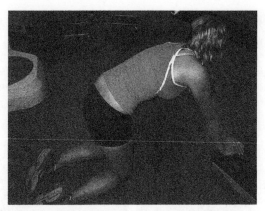

Fig. 7. Closed-chain step-up exercise for serratus anterior activation.

scapular musculature, and provide guidance to closed-chain exercise progression in the upper extremity.

ROTATOR CUFF STRENGTHENING

Strengthening the posterior rotator cuff to increase strength, fatigue resistance, and optimal muscle balance are emphasized when working with adolescent overhead athletes. **Fig. 8** shows the recommended exercises used by the authors for rotator cuff strengthening. These exercises are based on EMG research showing high levels of posterior rotator cuff activation.[48–51] Use of the prone horizontal abduction exercise is emphasized because research has shown this position to create high levels of supraspinatus muscular activation,[50,51] making it an alternative to the widely used empty can exercise that can cause impingement because of the combined inherent movements of internal rotation and elevation. Three sets of 15 to 20 repetitions are recommended to create a fatigue response and improve local muscular endurance.[52] For application to the patient with the initial levels of acute elbow pain, these exercises can be modified and performed using a cuff weight attached proximal to the elbow if distal weight attachment provokes pain or stresses the healing elbow structures. Moncreif and colleagues[53] have shown the efficacy of these exercises in a 4-week training paradigm and measured 8% to 10% increases in isokinetically measured internal and external rotation strength in healthy subjects. These isotonic exercises are coupled with an external rotation exercise with elastic resistance to provide resistance to the posterior rotator cuff in both a neutral and 90° abducted position in the scapular plane.

Carter and colleagues[54] studied the effects of an 8-week training program of plyometric upper extremity exercise and external rotation strengthening with elastic resistance. They found increased eccentric external rotation strength, concentric internal rotation strength, and improved throwing velocity in collegiate baseball players, showing the positive effects of plyometric and elastic resistance training in overhead athletes. **Fig. 9** shows a prone 90/90 plyometric that can be used with the athlete maintaining a retracted scapular position with the shoulder in 90° of abduction and 90° of external rotation. The plyo ball is rapidly dropped and caught over a 3- to 6-cm (2- to 3-inch) movement distance for sets of 30 to as much as 40 seconds to address local muscular endurance. Small 0.5 kg (1 pound) medicine balls or soft weights (Theraband; Hygenic Corporation Akron, OH, USA) are used initially, with progression to up to 1 kg as the adolescent patient progresses in both skill and strength development.

1. SIDELYING EXTERNAL ROTATION:
Lie on uninvolved side, with involved arm
at side, with a small pillow between arm
and body. Keeping elbow of involved arm bent
and fixed to side, raise arm into external
rotation. Slowly lower to starting position
and repeat.

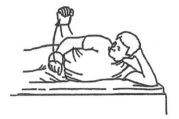

2. SHOULDER EXTENSION:
Lie on table on stomach, with involved arm
hanging straight to the floor. With thumb
pointed outward, raise arm straight back into
extension toward your hip. Slowly lower
arm and repeat.

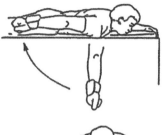

3. PRONE HORIZONTAL ABDUCTION:
Lie on table on stomach, with involved arm
hanging straight to the floor. With thumb
pointed outward, raise arm out to the side,
parallel to the floor. Slowly lower arm,
and repeat.

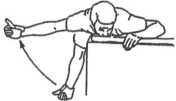

4. 90/90 EXTERNAL ROTATION:
Lie on table on stomach, with shoulder
abducted to 90 degrees and arm supported
on table, with elbow bent at 90 degrees.
Keeping the shoulder and elbow fixed,
rotate arm into external rotation, slowly
lower to start position, and repeat.

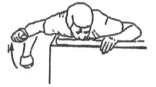

Fig. 8. Rotator cuff isotonic exercises. (*From* Ellenbecker TS, Pieczynski TE, Davies GJ. Rehabilitation of the elbow following sports injury. Clin Sports Med 2010;29:49; with permission.)

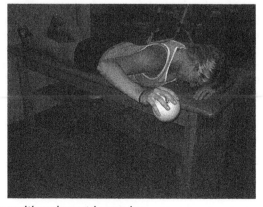

Fig. 9. 90/90 prone position plyometric exercise.

DISTAL UPPER EXTREMITY EXERCISES FOR THE ADOLESCENT OVERHEAD ATHLETE

Exercises to improve strength and promote muscular endurance of the forearm and wrist include both traditional curls for the flexors and extensors with either light isotonic dumbbells or elastic tubing or bands, as well as forearm pronation/supination and radioulnar deviation with a counterbalanced weight. These exercises help to provide additional muscular support to the distal extremity and provide protection and countering to the large forces encountered in this region with both throwing and overhead serving motions.

Because of the anatomic orientation of the flexor carpi ulnaris and flexor digitorum superficialis overlaying the UCL, isotonic and stabilization activities for these muscles may assist in stabilizing the medial elbow in the overhead throwing athlete.[13] These isotonic exercises with light weights or elastic tubing or bands form the base program for distal strengthening and are used in a low-resistance, high-repetition format.[1,55] Early use of extension and supination–based exercise may be indicated for the throwing athlete with medially based elbow symptoms until modalities and rest result in less pain and inflammation, then allowing wrist flexion and forearm pronation exercise. Progression to more advanced, ballistic-type exercises can be recommended for the adolescent overhead athlete following elbow injury in the later stages. Rapid ball dribbling in sets of 30 seconds with a basketball or small Swiss Ball are recommended, both off the ground and in an elevated position off the wall.

THE ROLE OF GLENOHUMERAL JOINT RANGE OF MOTION IN REHABILITATION AND PREVENTION OF ELBOW INJURY

Glenohumeral joint range of motion must also be monitored in the adolescent overhead athlete. Prior research has consistently shown increases in dominant arm external rotation and decreased internal rotation range of motion in adolescent throwers[56] and in elite junior tennis players.[57–59] Despite the bilateral difference in internal and external rotation, the total rotation range of motion (obtained by adding the internal and external rotation measures) was equal in the baseball players[56] and within 10° of the contralateral side in the elite tennis players. Dines and colleagues[60] have shown an association between UCL injury and glenohumeral joint internal rotation loss (glenohumeral internal rotation deficit [GIRD]). Based on these studies, it is recommended that any rehabilitation and/or prevention program for the adolescent overhead athlete should include both assessment of glenohumeral joint internal, external, and total rotation range of motion as well as treatment strategies to address internal rotation range of motion loss. McClure and colleagues[61] studied the effects of 2 stretches used to improve glenohumeral joint internal rotation range of motion in a prospective fashion. The stretches used and recommended in this study were the cross-arm stretch (**Fig. 10**), and sleeper stretches (**Fig. 11**), which both produced favorable increases in glenohumeral joint internal rotation during the 4-week study period. These stretches can be recommended for the adolescent overhead athlete to improve and maintain optimal glenohumeral joint internal rotation range of motion.

USE OF INTERVAL TENNIS AND THROWING PROGRAMS FOR THE ADOLESCENT OVERHEAD ATHLETE

One of the most often overlooked and underemphasized aspects of the rehabilitation process following elbow injury is the return to activity phase or interval return program, which can result in reinjury and delay an effective return to throwing or tennis performance. Objective criteria for entry into this stage are listed in **Box 1**.

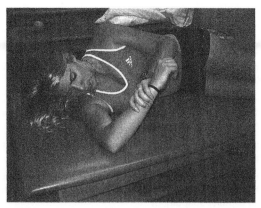

Fig. 10. Sleeper stretch.

Characteristics of interval sport return programs include alternate day performance, as well as gradual progressions of intensity and repetitions of sport activities. For the interval tennis program, for example, the initial use of a foam ball, progressing to a series of low-compression tennis balls such as the Pro-Penn Star Ball (Penn Racquet Sports, Phoenix, AZ, USA) both used during the teaching process of tennis to young children are recommended and followed (**Fig. 12**). These balls are recommended during the initial phase of the return to tennis program and are believed to result in

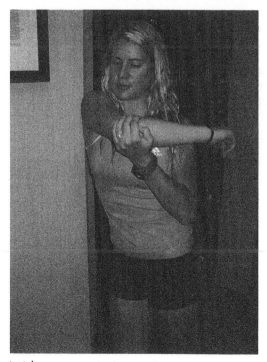

Fig. 11. Cross-arm stretch.

Box 1
Objective criterion recommended before progression to an interval return program following elbow injury in the overhead athlete

- Pain-free tolerance of the previously stated resistive exercise progressions for the scapula, rotator cuff, and distal upper extremity musculature

- Objective documentation of rotator cuff and wrist and forearm strength at a minimum level equal to the contralateral extremity with either manual assessment, hand-held dynamometry, or isokinetic testing

- Grip strength measured with a dynamometer equal to or greater than the contralateral side with no pain provocation

- Functional range of elbow, wrist, and forearm motion; in the elite athlete with musculoskeletal adaptations, full elbow range of motion is not always attainable, secondary to the osseous and capsular adaptations

---

a decrease in impact stress and increased patient tolerance to the early tennis-specific activity. Performing the interval program under supervision, either during physical therapy or with a knowledgeable tennis teaching professional or coach, allows for the biomechanical evaluation of technique and guards against overzealous intensity levels, which can be a common mistake in well-intentioned, motivated patients, especially adolescents. Using the return program on alternate days, with rest between sessions, allows for recovery and decreases the risk of reinjury.

An interval tennis program has been published[1,17] and a modified version is included as Appendix 1 in this article. It includes updated information on the use of the different tennis ball progressions and takes the player through a series progressing from groundstrokes to volleys and finally serves and overheads.

Similar concepts are used in the interval throwing program that was published previously.[62] Similarly to the interval tennis program, having the patient's throwing mechanics evaluated using video and by a qualified coach or biomechanist are important parts of the return to activity phase of the rehabilitation process. Integrating the program with physical therapy, or under the auspices of a knowledgeable coach, is recommended.

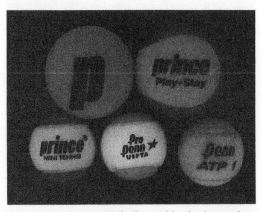

Fig. 12. Foam and low-compression tennis balls used in the interval tennis program.

SUMMARY

The concepts reviewed in this paper are important parts of the overall rehabilitation of an elbow injury in an adolescent overhead athlete. The exercise progressions and return to activity programs are integral parts of rehabilitation following an elbow injury. The exercise progressions outlined form an important part of a prevention program vital for elite level overhead athletes and, coupled with responsible programming, form the basis for injury prevention in this population of athletes.

APPENDIX 1: INTERVAL TENNIS PROGRAM

Interval tennis program guidelines

Begin at a stage indicated by your physical therapist or doctor

Do not progress or continue program if joint pain is present

Always stretch your shoulder, elbow, and wrist before and after the interval program, and perform a whole-body dynamic warm-up before performing the interval tennis program

Play on alternate days, giving your body a recovery day between sessions

Do not use a wall board or back board because it leads to exaggerated muscle contraction without rest between strokes. Ball feeds or ball machines are preferred

Ice your injured arm after each session of the interval tennis program

It is highly recommended to have your stroke mechanics formally evaluated by a US Professional Tennis Association tennis teaching professional

Do not attempt to impart heavy topspin or underspin to your groundstrokes until later in the interval program

Contact your therapist or doctor if you have questions or problems with the interval program

Do not continue to play if you encounter localized joint pain.

Interval tennis program:

Perform each stage a predetermined number of times before progressing to the next stage. Do not progress to the next stage if you have pain or excessive fatigue on your previous outing; remain at the previous stage until you can perform that part of the program without fatigue or pain.

Stage1

1. Have a partner feed 20 forehand groundstrokes to you from the net using a foam ball (partner must use a slow, looping feed that results in a waist-high ball bounce for player contact)
2. Have a partner feed 20 backhand groundstrokes, as in (a), with a foam ball
3. Rest 5 minutes
4. Repeat 20 forehand and backhand feeds as in (a) and (b).

Stage 2

Repeat stage 1 with a low-compression ball (ie, Pro-Penn Star Ball, Penn Racquet Sports, Phoenix, AZ, USA).

Stage 3

Repeat stage 1 with a real (regulation) tennis ball.

Stage 4

1. Begin as in stage 3, with partner feeding 10 forehands and 10 backhands from the net as a warm-up

2. Rally with partner from baseline, hitting controlled groundstrokes until you have hit 50 to 60 strokes (alternate between forehands and backhands and allow 20–30 seconds rest after every 2–3 rallies)
3. Rest 5 minutes
4. Repeat the rally instructions in (b).

Stage 5
1. Rally groundstrokes (forehands and backhands) from the baseline for 15 minutes
2. Rest 5 minutes
3. Hit 10 to 15 forehand and 10 to 15 backhand volleys, emphasizing a contact point in front of your body
4. Rally groundstrokes for 15 additional minutes from the baseline
5. Hit 10 to 15 forehand and backhand volleys as in (c).

Preserve interval: (perform before stage 6)
(Note: this interval can be performed off court and is meant solely to determine readiness for progression into stage 6 of the interval tennis program)
1. After stretching, with racquet in hand, perform serving motion for 10 to 15 repetitions without a ball or any ball contact
2. Using a foam ball, hit 10 to 15 serves without concern for performance result (only focusing on form, contact point, and the presence or absence of symptoms)
3. If successful and pain free, progress to stage 6.

Stage 6
1. Hit 20 to 30 minutes of groundstrokes, mixing in volleys using an 80% groundstroke/20% volley format
2. Perform 5 to 10 simulated serves without a ball
3. Perform 5 to 10 serves using a foam ball
4. Perform 10 to 15 serves using a standard tennis ball at approximately 75% effort (it is important to hit flat or slice serves, not kick serves, in the initial phase of the interval tennis program)
5. Finish with 10 to 15 minutes of groundstrokes.

Stage 7
1. Hit 30 minutes of groundstrokes, mixing in volleys using an 80% groundstroke/20% volley format
2. Perform 5 to 10 serves using a foam ball
3. Perform 10 to 15 serves using a standard tennis ball at approximately 75% effort
4. Rest 5 minutes
5. Perform 10 to 15 additional serves as in (c)
6. Finish with 15 to 20 minutes of groundstrokes.

Stage 8
1. Repeat stage 7, increasing the number of serves to 20 or 25 instead of 10 or 15
2. Before resting between serving sessions, have a partner feed easy short lobs to attempt 4 to 5 controlled overheads.

Stage 9
Before attempting match play, complete steps 1 to 8 without pain or excess fatigue in the upper extremity. Continue to progress the amount of time rallying with groundstrokes and volleys in addition to increasing the number of serves per workout until 60 to 80 overall serves can be performed, interspersed throughout a workout. Initiate kick serves once the initial stages of the program have been completed. Remember that an

average of up to 120 serves can be performed in a singles tennis match, so be prepared to gradually increase the number of serves in the interval program before full competitive play is engaged.

APPENDIX 2: INTERVAL THROWING PROGRAM FOR ADOLESCENT BASEBALL PLAYERS

30-ft Phase	45-ft Phase
Step 1:	Step 3:
(A) Warm-up throwing	(A) Warm-up throwing
(B) 30 ft (25 throws)	(B) 45 ft (25 throws)
(C) Rest 15 min	(C) Rest 15 min
(D) Warm-up throwing	(D) Warm-up throwing
(E) 30 ft (25 throws)	(E) 45 ft (25 throws)
Step 2:	Step 4:
(A) Warm-up throwing	(A) Warm-up throwing
(B) 30 ft (25 throws)	(B) 45 ft (25 throws)
(C) Rest 10 min	(C) Rest 10 min
(D) Warm-up throwing	(D) Warm-up throwing
(E) 30 ft (25 throws)	(E) 45 ft (25 throws)
(F) Rest 10 min	(F) Rest 10 min
(G) Warm-up throwing	(G) Warm-up throwing
(H) 30 ft (25 throws)	(H) 45 ft (25 throws)
60-ft Phase	**90-ft Phase**
Step 5:	Step 7:
(A) Warm-up throwing	(A) Warm-up throwing
(B) 60 ft (25 throws)	(B) 90 ft (25 throws)
(C) Rest 15 min	(C) Rest 15 min
(D) Warm-up throwing	(D) Warm-up throwing
(E) 60 ft (25 throws)	(E) 90 ft (25 throws)
Step 6:	Step 8:
(A) Warm-up throwing	(A) Warm-up throwing
(B) 60 ft (25 throws)	(B) 90 ft (20 throws)
(C) Rest 10 min	(C) Rest 10 min
(D) Warm-up throwing	(D) Warm-up throwing
(E) 60 ft (25 throws)	(E) 60 ft (20 throws)
(F) Rest 10 min	(F) Rest 10 min
(G) Warm-up throwing	(G) Warm-up throwing
(H) 60 ft (25 throws)	(H) 45 ft (20 throws)
	(I) Rest 10 min
	(J) Warm-up throwing
	(K) 45 ft (15 throws)

30 ft = 9.1 m, 45 ft = 13.7 m, 60 ft = 18.3 m, 90 ft = 27.4 m.

REFERENCES

1. Ellenbecker TS, Mattalino AJ. The elbow in sport. Champaign (IL): Human Kinetics Publishers; 1997.
2. Lyman S, Fleisig GS, Andrews JR, et al. Effect of pitch type, pitch count, and pitching mechanics on risk of elbow and shoulder pain in youth baseball pitchers. Am J Sports Med 2002;30:463–8.
3. Auvinen JP, Tammelin TH, Taimela SP, et al. Musculoskeletal pains in relation to different sport and exercise activities in youth. Med Sci Sports Exerc 2008;40(11):1890–900.

4. Albright JA, Jokl P, Shaw R, et al. Clinical study of baseball pitchers: correlation of injury to the throwing arm with method of delivery. Am J Sports Med 1978;6: 15–21.
5. Grana WA, Rashkin A. Pitcher's elbow in adolescents. Am J Sports Med 1980;8: 333–6.
6. Hang YS, Lippett FG, Spolek GH, et al. Biomechanical study of the pitching elbow. Int Orthop 1979;3(3):217–23.
7. Lyman S, Fleisig GS, Waterbor JW, et al. Longitudinal study of elbow and shoulder pain in youth baseball pitchers. Med Sci Sports Exerc 2001;33(11): 1803–10.
8. Dun S, Loftice J, Fleisig GS, et al. A biomechanical comparison of youth baseball pitches: is the curveball potentially harmful? Am J Sports Med 2008;36: 686–92.
9. Nissen CW, Westwell M, Ounpuu S, et al. A biomechanical comparison of the fastball and curveball in adolescent baseball pitchers. Am J Sports Med 2009; 37:1492–8.
10. Fleisig GS, Kinglsey DS, Loftice JW, et al. Kinetic comparison among the fastball, curveball, change-up and slider in collegiate baseball pitchers. Am J Sports Med 2006;34:423–30.
11. Fleisig GS, Andrews JR, Dillman CJ, et al. Kinetics of baseball pitching with implications about injury mechanisms. Am J Sports Med 1995;23:233–9.
12. Seiber K, Gupta R, McGarry MH, et al. The role of the elbow musculature, forearm rotation, and elbow flexion in elbow stability: an in-vitro study. J Shoulder Elbow Surg 2009;18(2):260–8.
13. Davidson PA, Pink M, Perry J, et al. Functional anatomy of the flexor pronator muscle group in relation to the medial collateral ligament of the elbow. Am J Sports Med 1995;23(2):245–50.
14. An KN, Fui HC, Morrey BF, et al. Muscles that cross the elbow joint: a biomechanical analysis. J Biomech 1981;14(10):659–69.
15. Olsen SJ 2nd, Fleisig GS, Dun S, et al. Risk factors for shoulder and elbow injuries in adolescent baseball pitchers. Am J Sports Med 2006;34(6):905–12.
16. Davis JT, Limpisvasti O, Fluhme D, et al. The effect of pitching biomechanics on the upper extremity in youth and adolescent baseball pitchers. Am J Sports Med 2009;37:1484–91.
17. Ellenbecker TS. Rehabilitation of shoulder and elbow injuries in tennis players. Clin Sports Med 1995;14(1):87–110.
18. Johnson CD, McHugh MP. Performance demands of professional male tennis players. Br J Sports Med 2006;40:696–9.
19. Kibler WB. Clinical biomechanics of the elbow in tennis. Implications for evaluation and diagnosis. Med Sci Sports Exerc 1994;26:1203–6.
20. Morris M, Jobe FW, Perry J, et al. Electromyographic analysis of elbow function in the tennis players. Am J Sports Med 1989;17:241–7.
21. Ryu KN, McCormick J, Jobe FW, et al. An electromyographic analysis of shoulder function in tennis players. Am J Sports Med 1988;16:481–5.
22. Wilson FD, Andrews JR, Blackburn TA, et al. Valgus extension overload in pitching elbow. Am J Sports Med 1983;11:83–8.
23. Indelicato PA, Jobe FW, Kerlan RK, et al. Correctable elbow lesions in professional baseball players: a review of 25 cases. Am J Sports Med 1979;7:72–5.
24. Elliott BC, Mester J, Kleinoder H, et al. Loading and stroke production. In: Elliott BC, Reid M, Crespo M, editors. Biomechanics of advanced tennis. London: International Tennis Federation; 2003.

25. Segal DK. Tenis sistema biodinamico. Buenos Aires (Argentina): Tenis Club Argentino; 2002.
26. ITF. London (United Kingdom): International Tennis Federation; 2009.
27. Kovacs M, Ellenbecker TS, Kibler WB, et al. Demographic data and potential trends in competitive American junior tennis. Society of Tennis Medicine and Science (STMS) World Conference. Valencia (Spain), November 10, 2009.
28. Reece LA, Fricker PA, Maguire KA. Injuries to elite young tennis players at the Australian Institute of Sports. Aust J Sci Med Sport 1986;18:11–5.
29. Kibler WB, McQueen C, Uhl T. Fitness evaluation and fitness findings in competitive junior tennis players. Clin Sports Med 1988;7:403–16.
30. Giangarra CE, Conroy B, Jobe FW, et al. Electromyographic and cinematographic analysis of elbow function in tennis players using single- and double-handed backhand strokes. Am J Sports Med 1993;21:394–9.
31. Chen FR, Diaz VA, Loebenberg M, et al. Shoulder and elbow injuries in the skeletally immature athlete. J Am Acad Orthop Surg 2005;13:172–85.
32. Hang DW, Chao CM, Hang YS. A clinical and roentgenographic study of Little League elbow. Am J Sports Med 2004;32:79–84.
33. Kobayashi K, Burton KJ, Rodner C, et al. Lateral compression injuries in the pediatric elbow: Panner's disease and osteochondritis dissecans of the capitellum. J Am Acad Orthop Surg 2004;12:246–54.
34. Ahmad CS, ElAttrache NS. Valgus extension overload syndrome and stress injury of the olecranon. Clin Sports Med 2004;23:665–76.
35. Davies GJ, Ellenbecker TS. The scientific and clinical rationale for the utilization of a total arm strength rehabilitation program for shoulder and elbow overuse injury, orthopaedic home study course. LaCrosse (WI): American Physical Therapy Association; 1992.
36. Kibler WB. Role of the scapula in the overhead throwing motion. Contemp Orthop 1991;22(5):525–32.
37. Kibler WB. The role of the scapula in athletic shoulder function. Am J Sports Med 1998;26(2):325–37.
38. Inman VT, Saunders JB, Abbott LC. Observations on the function of the shoulder joint. J Bone Joint Surg 1944;26(1):1–30.
39. Kibler WB, Uhl TL, Maddux JW, et al. Qualitative clinical evaluation of scapular dysfunction: a reliability study. J Shoulder Elbow Surg 2002;11:550–6.
40. Tate AR, McClure P, Kareha S, et al. A clinical method for identifying scapular dyskinesis, part 2: validity. J Athl Train 2009;44(2):165–73.
41. McClure P, Tate AR, Kareha S, et al. A clinical method for identifying scapular dyskinesis, part 1: reliability. J Athl Train 2009;44(2):160–4.
42. Ellenbecker TS, Kibler WB, Bailie, et al. Interrater reliability of a scapular classification system in the musculoskeletal examination of professional baseball players [abstract]. J Orthop Sports Phys Ther 2008;39:A108.
43. McCabe RA, Orishimo KF, McHugh MP, et al. Surface electromyographic analysis of the lower trapezius muscle during exercises performed below ninety degrees of shoulder elevation in healthy subject. N Am J Sports Phys Ther 2007;2(1):34–43.
44. Kibler WB, Sciascia AD, Uhl TL, et al. Electromyographic analysis of specific exercises for scapular control in early phases of shoulder rehabilitation. Am J Sports Med 2008;36:1789–98.
45. Moseley JB, Jobe FW, Pink M. EMG analysis of the scapular muscles during a shoulder rehabilitation program. Am J Sports Med 1992;20:128–34.
46. Decker MJ, Hintermeister RA, Faber KJ, et al. Serratus anterior muscle activity during selected rehabilitation exercises. Am J Sports Med 1999;27:784–91.

47. Uhl TL, Carver TJ, Mattacola CG, et al. Shoulder musculature activation during upper extremity weightbearing exercise. J Orthop Sports Phys Ther 2003;33(3): 109–17.
48. Ballantyne BT, O'Hare SJ, Paschall JL, et al. Electromyographic activity of selected shoulder muscles in commonly used therapeutic exercises. Phys Ther 1993;73:668–77.
49. Blackburn TA, McLeod WD, White B, et al. EMG analysis of posterior rotator cuff exercises. Athletic Training 1990;25:40–5.
50. Reinhold MM, Wilk KE, Fleisig GS, et al. Electromyographic analysis of the rotator cuff and deltoid musculature during common shoulder external rotation exercises. J Orthop Sports Phys Ther 2004;34:385–94.
51. Townsend H, Jobe FW, Pink M, et al. Electromyographic analysis of the glenohumeral muscles during a baseball rehabilitation program. Am J Sports Med 1991;19:264–72.
52. Fleck SJ, Kraemer WJ. Designing resistance training programs. Champaign (IL): Human Kinetics Publishers; 1987.
53. Moncrief SA, Lau JD, Gale JR, et al. Effect of rotator cuff exercise on humeral rotation torque in healthy individuals. J Strength Cond Res 2002;16:262–70.
54. Carter AB, Kaminsky TW, Douex T Jr, et al. Effects of high volume upper extremity plyometric training on throwing velocity and functional strength ratios of the shoulder rotators in collegiate baseball players. J Strength Cond Res 2007;21(1):208–15.
55. Ellenbecker TS, Wilk KE, Altchek DW, et al. Current concepts in rehabilitation following ulnar collateral ligament reconstruction. Sports Health 2009;1:301–13.
56. Meister K, Day T, Horodyski MB, et al. Rotational motion changes in the glenohumeral joint of the adolescent Little League baseball player. Am J Sports Med 2005;33:693–8.
57. Ellenbecker TS. Shoulder internal and external rotation strength and range of motion in highly skilled tennis players. Isokinet Exerc Sci 1992;2:1–8.
58. Ellenbecker TS, Roetert EP, Piorkowski PA. Shoulder internal and external rotation range of motion of elite junior tennis players: a comparison of two protocols. J Orthop Sports Phys Ther 1993;17:65.
59. Ellenbecker TS, Roetert EP, Bailie DS, et al. Glenohumeral joint total rotation range of motion in elite tennis players and baseball pitchers. Med Sci Sports Exerc 2002;34:2052–6.
60. Dines JS, Frank JB, Akerman M, et al. Glenohumeral internal rotation deficits in baseball players with ulnar collateral ligament deficiency. Am J Sports Med 2009;37(3):566–70.
61. McClure P, Balaicuis J, Heiland D, et al. A randomized controlled comparison of stretching procedures for posterior shoulder tightness. J Orthop Sports Phys Ther 2007;37:108–14.
62. Reinold MM, Wilk KE, Reed J, et al. Interval sport programs: guidelines for baseball, tennis, and golf. J Orthop Sports Phys Ther 2002;32:293–8.

Index

Note: Page numbers of article titles are in **boldface** type.

Clin Sports Med 29 (2010) 725–731
doi:10.1016/S0278-5919(10)00069-4
0278-5919/10/$ – see front matter © 2010 Elsevier Inc. All rights reserved.

sportsmed.theclinics.com

Moving?

Make sure your subscription moves with you!

To notify us of your new address, find your **Clinics Account Number** (located on your mailing label above your name), and contact customer service at:

Email: journalscustomerservice-usa@elsevier.com

800-654-2452 (subscribers in the U.S. & Canada)
314-447-8871 (subscribers outside of the U.S. & Canada)

Fax number: 314-447-8029

Elsevier Health Sciences Division
Subscription Customer Service
3251 Riverport Lane
Maryland Heights, MO 63043

United States Postal Service

Statement of Ownership, Management, and Circulation
(All Periodicals Publications Except Requester Publications)

1. Publication Title	2. Publication Number	3. Filing Date
Clinics in Sports Medicine	0 0 0 - 7 0 2	9/15/10

4. Issue Frequency	5. Number of Issues Published Annually	6. Annual Subscription Price
Jan, Apr, Jul, Oct	4	$278.00

7. Complete Mailing Address of Known Office of Publication (Not printer) (Street, city, county, state, and ZIP+4®)

Elsevier Inc.
360 Park Avenue South
New York, NY 10010-1710

Contact Person
Stephen Bushing
Telephone (Include area code)
215-239-3688

8. Complete Mailing Address of Headquarters or General Business Office of Publisher (Not printer)

Elsevier Inc., 360 Park Avenue South, New York, NY 10010-1710

9. Full Names and Complete Mailing Addresses of Publisher, Editor, and Managing Editor (Do not leave blank)

Publisher (Name and complete mailing address)

Kim Murphy, Elsevier, Inc., 1600 John F. Kennedy Blvd. Suite 1800, Philadelphia, PA 19103-2899

Editor (Name and complete mailing address)

Ruth Malwitz, Elsevier, Inc., 1600 John F. Kennedy Blvd. Suite 1800, Philadelphia, PA 19103-2899

Managing Editor (Name and complete mailing address)

Catherine Bewick, Elsevier, Inc., 1600 John F. Kennedy Blvd. Suite 1800, Philadelphia, PA 19103-2899

10. Owner (Do not leave blank. If the publication is owned by a corporation, give the name and address of the corporation immediately followed by the names and addresses of all stockholders owning or holding 1 percent or more of the total amount of stock. If not owned by a corporation, give the names and addresses of the individual owners. If owned by a partnership or other unincorporated firm, give its name and address as well as those of each individual owner. If the publication is published by a nonprofit organization, give its name and address.)

Full Name	Complete Mailing Address
Wholly owned subsidiary of	4520 East-West Highway
Reed/Elsevier, US holdings	Bethesda, MD 20814

11. Known Bondholders, Mortgagees, and Other Security Holders Owning or Holding 1 Percent or More of Total Amount of Bonds, Mortgages, or Other Securities. If none, check box ☐ None

Full Name	Complete Mailing Address
N/A	

12. Tax Status (For completion by nonprofit organizations authorized to mail at nonprofit rates) (Check one)
The purpose, function, and nonprofit status of this organization and the exempt status for federal income tax purposes:
☐ Has Not Changed During Preceding 12 Months
☐ Has Changed During Preceding 12 Months (Publisher must submit explanation of change with this statement)

PS Form 3526, September 2007 (Page 1 of 3 (Instructions Page 3)) PSN 7530-01-000-9931 PRIVACY NOTICE: See our Privacy policy in www.usps.com

---

13. Publication Title	14. Issue Date for Circulation Data Below
Clinics in Sports Medicine	July 2010

15. Extent and Nature of Circulation		Average No. Copies Each Issue During Preceding 12 Months	No. Copies of Single Issue Published Nearest to Filing Date
a. Total Number of Copies (Net press run)		1561	1428
b. Paid Circulation (By Mail and Outside the Mail)	(1) Mailed Outside-County Paid Subscriptions Stated on PS Form 3541. (Include paid distribution above nominal rate, advertiser's proof copies, and exchange copies)	807	770
	(2) Mailed In-County Paid Subscriptions Stated on PS Form 3541 (Include paid distribution above nominal rate, advertiser's proof copies, and exchange copies)		
	(3) Paid Distribution Outside the Mails Including Sales Through Dealers and Carriers, Street Vendors, Counter Sales, and Other Paid Distribution Outside USPS®	217	177
	(4) Paid Distribution by Other Classes Mailed Through the USPS (e.g. First-Class Mail®)		
c. Total Paid Distribution (Sum of 15b (1), (2), (3), and (4))	▶	1024	947
d. Free or Nominal Rate Distribution (By Mail and Outside the Mail)	(1) Free or Nominal Rate Outside-County Copies Included on PS Form 3541	89	76
	(2) Free or Nominal Rate In-County Copies Included on PS Form 3541		
	(3) Free or Nominal Rate Copies Mailed at Other Classes Through the USPS (e.g. First-Class Mail)		
	(4) Free or Nominal Rate Distribution Outside the Mail (Carriers or other means)		
e. Total Free or Nominal Rate Distribution (Sum of 15d (1), (2), (3) and (4))	▶	89	76
f. Total Distribution (Sum of 15c and 15e)	▶	1113	1023
g. Copies not Distributed (See instructions to publishers #4 (page #3))	▶	448	405
h. Total (Sum of 15f and g)	▶	1561	1428
i. Percent Paid (15c divided by 15f times 100)	▶	92.00%	92.57%

16. Publication of Statement of Ownership

☐ If the publication is a general publication, publication of this statement is required. Will be printed in the October 2010 issue of this publication. ☐ Publication not required

17. Signature and Title of Editor, Publisher, Business Manager, or Owner

Stephen R. Bushing — Fulfillment/Inventory Specialist

	Date
Stephen R. Bushing – Fulfillment/Inventory Specialist	September 15, 2010

I certify that all information furnished on this form is true and complete. I understand that anyone who furnishes false or misleading information on this form or who omits material or information requested on the form may be subject to criminal sanctions (including fines and imprisonment) and/or civil sanctions (including civil penalties).

PS Form 3526, September 2007 (Page 2 of 3)